Green Is 4 Life:

A Simple Guide To Creating Healthy Life-Giving Green Smoothies

Green Is 4 Life:

A Simple Guide To Creating
Healthy Life-Giving Green Smoothies

Dr. Wendy Dearborne

First Edition
First publishing, 2013

Editor Bonita Kale

Dr. Wendy Dearborne may be contacted at 2770 S. Maryland Pkwy #307, Las Vegas, Nevada 89109 Telephone 702.425.8589 Visit her websites www.itsmylifemychoice.com and www.drwendydearborne.com

Note to Reader
This book has been written and published strictly for informational and educational purposes. It is not intended to serve as medical advice or to be any form of medical treatment. You should always consult your physician before altering and changing any aspect of your medical treatment and or undertaking a diet regimen, including green smoothie fasting and green smoothie inclusion guidelines described in this book.

Do not stop or change any prescription medication without the guidance and advice of your physician. Any information from this book is to be used based on the reader's good judgment after consulting with his or her physician and is the reader's sole responsibility. This book is not intended to diagnose or treat any medical condition and is not a substitute for a physician or health care professional.

DEDICATION

This book is for people all over the globe who have made the choice to take a proactive approach to their health care through diet and nutrition. It's for all who feel disenfranchised and powerless to create healthy eating lifestyles and are challenged by adding fresh fruits and vegetables to their diet. It's for all people who don't want to be told what they can't or shouldn't eat, but told what they can include into their current diets, to support and create a healthier way of living.

CONTENTS

PREFACE

Green Is 4 Life: A Simple Guide To Creating Life-Giving Green Smoothies is not a treatise on nutrition. *Green Is 4 Life* is all about eating whole life-giving foods in a way that makes them easy to prepare and digest, which influences optimal health and integration of the mind, body, and spirit. You will not find within these chapters, reams of statistical information scientifically splintering apart this food or that food to isolate one nutritional component and tout it as the next great cure-all.

Green Is 4 Life is about choice. Namely *your* choice—how you choose to influence your health and subsequently your existence through eating live, whole, green leafy vegetables, other vegetables, nuts, seeds, grains, fresh fruit and water.

Green Is 4 Life is not another fad diet book. It's a book all about the inclusion of life-giving raw foods into your current lifestyle in the form of a delicious green smoothie. The pages within this book are not about deprivation or the exclusion of things that you currently love and want to continue eating.

Green Is 4 Life is about inclusion, not exclusion—the inclusion of life-giving live foods into your current dietary practice. You will not be inundated with numerous recipes designed for calorie counting, fats to avoid, or carbs to eat or not to eat. Neither will you find any statistical information. You can find all the statistical, scientific, and nutritional data on what various foods outlined in this book are reported and purported to do, online or in your local bookstore and/or local library.

The reason I have elected not to add any statistical data is really very simple: *I believe that, whenever possible, it's important to use your own personal experience, and not someone else's, to support and assist you in your choice-making process. I call it "doing your own due diligence."* Be prepared, because you will hear, *"Do your own due diligence,"* and, *"Start where you are at,"* over and over throughout this book. *Start where you are at,* literally means *start* with whatever you have on hand. Or making purchases that do not take you outside of your financial comfort zone.

ACKNOWLEDGMENTS

I give thanks for all the choices that I have made, the good the bad and the in-between, for each and every choice has made me who I am. And for the eternal flame that burns brightly within me that inspires me to want to inspire others, I give thanks.

To my husband, Eddie Lee "Dee" Dearborne, without whose love, care, wisdom, and support, much of what I have accomplished might have taken me several lifetimes. Thank you for loving me!

To Expression Coach and Artist Olivia Lashley, my youngest sister, thank you for being my sounding board and encouraging me when I felt like giving up. And to my Mum who made me believe that I could do and be anything I chose to be, and my Dad who taught me to question life and for generously allowing me a month of solitude so that I could write to my heart's content. To my sister's Gina and Joan who made me believe that I can. To my brother "Penny" who taught me to stand upon my word. And, to Tracy Kaelin for the Vitamix fund.

To my loyal and loving clients, your support means so much to me.

v

My eternal gratitude goes to Dr. Bonita Kale, for skillfully editing my manuscript, yet keeping the voice authentically me. Thank you so much!

I give thanks for the profound insight, wisdom, and motivation that the following words have imparted into my life: "From your cradle to your grave everything in between is created by your choice."

I've heard it said that the most important thing written on your headstone is not your name or your age. It's not even the celebration of your birth or the mourning of your death, but it's the dash in between your date of birth and the date of your death. That, little dash, that small hyphen in between, represents your life and all the choices that you have made. So, create the life that you want to live through the power of your conscious choice.

To Rosemarie Jennifer, until we meet again...thank you Sis and I love you much.

INTRODUCTION
HOW TO USE GREEN IS 4 LIFE

This book takes a straightforward, no-nonsense look at adding nutritional value to our diets with the intention of improving the quality of our lives, by blending and adding raw green leafy vegetables, vegetables, fruits and nut, seed and grain milks.

Green Is 4 Life has been written to support and assist anyone who wants definitive information on the nuts and bolts of green smoothie fasting and/or including green smoothies into their current dietary lifestyle.

This book has been written for people all over the globe who have made the choice to take a proactive approach to their health care through the inclusion of the nutrients and micronutrients found in eating whole, live, raw, fresh foods.

It's for all whom feel disenfranchised and powerless to create healthy eating habits and are challenged by incorporating fresh fruits and vegetables into their diet. It's for people who don't want to be told what they can't or shouldn't eat, but told what they can add to their diets to support and create healthier lifestyles. It's for you!

The chapters in this book offer you several concepts. The first is that, as all our lives are built one choice at a time, it's important that I— you—we — create and compile our own statistical information, about things that pertain to each of us. It's imperative not to base all your decisions on what others perceive to be true for them, thus making it an ironclad truth for you. Remember that sage old adage, "One man's meat is another man's poison."

Second, with those words in mind, in regard to whatever you read within the pages of this book, I humbly suggest doing your own due diligence. Let your experience speak for itself, so that you can make informed choices about your life.

Third, here are the nuts and bolts of adding fresh fruits and vegetables, in particular green, leafy vegetables, into your diet with ease and simplicity. You will also, learn one basic principle that can be applied to any dietary lifestyle. You will create life-giving food within every glass filled with a green smoothie.

And fourth, if green smoothies are not for you, I'll show how to add life-giving fresh vegetables to your dinner plate.

For tips and suggestions, checkout the questions and answers at the end of each chapter.

PART ONE

CHAPTER 1
LIFE IS BUILT ONE CHOICE AT A TIME

The amazing life that we are currently living is built, one miraculous choice at a time. Each choice we have made, has acted as the foundation for what is happening in our lives NOW, in this moment. And, perhaps more importantly, the choices we are going to make will be the building blocks for the life we aspire to live. How we choose to feel about the outcome of our choices denotes whether we perceive them as good or bad. The thing to remember is that, good or bad, happy or sad, you are in control of the choices you make in your life.

What you don't get to control is people's reactions to your choices. This is illustrated daily by the little and big things that people do or don't do in response to a choice you have made. Just as a stonemason or building contractor erects a house one brick or segment at a time, we erect our lives one choice at a time. The knowledge that one step, one choice, can create that which you want is empowering.

Experiencing empowerment, which may be called control and or feeling and maintaining an authentic sense of confidence about oneself, boils down to one thing: ownership of your choices!

Ownership of one's choices is synonymous with responsibility and accountability. To take control of and be proactive in your life, finances, careers, relationships and (as in my case) health, you have to OWN how you have arrived at this point, and you have to own how you are going to change it.

Now, owning how I came to the point of "dis-ease" in my life, for the second time where serious medical intervention was required, wasn't about delving into and dissecting my past behaviors. Although acknowledging past behaviors is and always will be important, it's not helpful to get mired down in the past. However, acknowledged past behaviors can help clarify and solidify the direction you want your life to take.

Ownership of my life was and is all about me and what I want for my health, both now and in the future. It is all about what it will look like for me to achieve it. How I saw this happening and what others, including doctors, saw, are, and will always remain two different things. You see, your life pertains to you, and, yes, other people will support and assist you. But the ultimate decision as to what you do belongs to you.

To create effective change in your life, you must first perceive, so that you can then conceive of what will give the inspiration and motivation to achieve it…whatever "it" is for you.

In my case, as you will read in the following pages of this book, I want to achieve what I consider to be optimal health for me. Not what someone else thought was right for me, but what I, Wendy, instinctively knew was right for me. I recognized that in order to do that, I had to make a conscious, committed choice to change things that I was currently doing in my life. I had to create a foundation with crystal-clear clarity.

Albert Einstein said, "Insanity: doing the same thing over and over again expecting different results."

And that was basically what I was doing and had been doing for a long time, a very long, long time. I'd been feeding myself a line of BS and the scary part was I believed my own hype. I was doing the same thing over and over again and expecting a different outcome. I know this because the outcome in our lives never lies. The outcome of my choices reflected the exact choices I had made. Otherwise, I would not have wound up back at a point that I had been at three decades ago.

It's Your Right to Be Healthy
It's your life; it's your choice

It's your birthright to be healthy. To maintain that birthright takes responsibility, accountability, and ownership of the choices that will reflect what you want for yourself.

On a fateful day in June 2011, the underlying thought I had running through my mind was, *It's my life; it's my choice,* along with an overwhelming sense of déjà vu, tinged with dread. These thoughts and feelings told me one thing: *Wendy, you've been this route before!* And this explained why I was feeling such a sense of suffocating dread. I had been here before.

You see, 31 years ago, almost to the day, I had been paraded before numerous doctors. Doctors! Doctors! Doctors! So many doctors, all gleefully humming and harring; a.k.a, hemming and hawing. Doctors squinting and poking, draining me of my precious, life-sustaining blood, all with the intent of diagnosing what was wrong with me.

On that fateful day, as I sat in the miserable, gray, and musty-smelling University Medical Center quick-care waiting room, depressed and a lot afraid, my inner self chose that moment to have a little tête-à-tête with me. As I couldn't run away from myself or the chatter inside my head, nor get into a shouting match with it, I elected to listen, sitting hunched over and dejected.

My Inner Self, which has always proved to date to be right, stated baldly, *"You know they're going to want to give you a steroid injection, along with oral steroids. Oh and, the M&M's of the pharmaceutical world, antibiotics, just for good measure."*

Because of my background and in conjunction with the nature of my complaint, which I'll get to in a second, I was in total, abject agreement. So much so that, at that point, I made the decision to refuse the steroid injection, if, and only if, they prescribed orals to go along with it. And of course, they would have to explain why I needed to take the antibiotic.

Q: Do I have control over my health?
A: Yes you do! Your health is a matter of choice…your choice.

So my question to you is what does it look like, feel like, sound like, taste like or smell like for you to be healthy? When you can answer that question, you'll be able to find your way to your optimal health. You'll be able to make choices in the best interest of your self. You be able to create baby steps or quantum leaps that will take you there.

CHAPTER 2
SO WHAT WAS WRONG WITH ME?

I had been experiencing a problem with my skin. Sometimes parts of my skin itched to the point that I felt like something was moving under my skin. Patches of skin would swell and sometimes present a cluster of wheals that would crack open and bleed.

It started out on my scalp and got so bad I was scratching my head bloody, which I knew could lead to permanent baldness. Being bald didn't coincide with my self-image, so I went to see two dermatologists. They didn't exactly give me a solid diagnosis. And of course, one prescribed a very expensive steroid shampoo and the other an equally expensive steroid lotion.

Hallelujah! I was doing the happy dance. You know the Tootsie Roll, Cabbage Patching, Second lining, Electric Sliding, and Crunking! It did the trick. Within 24 hours of using the shampoo, I experienced a noticeable difference with my scalp. The itching, burning, and of course the bleeding and hair loss, stopped. Just like that! Wow! It was magical…or so I thought.

Thirty-one years ago, I had taken large dosages of steroids for eighteen months to combat a disease called Sarcoidosis. Because of my understanding about the ramifications of steroid use, I became somewhat non-compliant. What can I say other than I am my mother's daughter? I only used the steroid based shampoo when things started to get out of control. About two years into this process, I noticed I had to use the shampoo more frequently. Then one day out of the blue the palms of my hands started to itch. The next thing I knew was that my right palm cracked open and started bleeding. As a reflexologist, facial therapist, and energy worker, I work with my hands touching people. Who wants to be touched by a cracked, bleeding hand? Not only was it unsightly that my skin was splitting open, but my first barrier of defense against any alien marauders wanting to invade my body was gone.

Somewhere in the recesses of my mind I recognized, but refused to acknowledge, that my problem might have become systemic. I sigh deeply here, because past experience, personal and professional, tells me that putting the lid on a pot of boiling water does not extinguish the flame under it.

I made the choice to use a combination of many of the healing arts that I am skilled at. Being a master aromatherapist, I decided to use the extensive knowledge that I already had, coupled with new research. (Incidentally, I'm having an illicit affair with the internet. I am in LOVE with a guy called Google and he is sooooooooooo in love with me.) With new-found knowledge in hand, I created several clinical essential-oil blends for this condition. (Not that I knew exactly what my condition was.) Anyway, the blends I created worked wonders for a while and of course, I was jazzed. I was healed. It was magical…or so I thought.

Then the bubble burst when the left palm and the backs of both hands developed the same condition. And all the while my scalp was getting worse and worse. "And you know this how Wendy?" Because I was using the steroid shampoo every other day. Plus I started using the creamy steroid lotion.

Systematically, areas over my body were being afflicted: my lower back and groin, my ankles and the soles of my feet. Also behind my ears, along my chin and on the outer edges of my nostrils. I was, to coin a phrase, "MESSED UP!"

But what really gave the game away and had me running to the nearest UMC Quick Care was that on June 15, 2011, my eyelids, upper and lower were almost swollen shut and I had multiple places where the lids had split open!

And to add insult to my already injured self, I couldn't get my contact lens out. (Yeah, I said, "contact lens" because I only have to wear one lens in my left eye…go figure.)

Long story short: the doctor at the UMC Quick care diagnosed me with having "possible allergies and possible contact dermatitis." I was offered the prerequisite steroid shot, which I grumpily declined. I was also given an oral prescription for prednisolone and antibiotics for my eyes. I did query the antibiotic thing. I was told by the attending physician, "This is a precautionary measure, just in case you have an infection in your eye."

I did take the prednisolone as prescribed, but elected not to use the antibiotic for my eyes. I didn't think that I had an eye infection...and I was right. Within two days of taking the steroids, everything calmed down. By Saturday, my skin looked fantastic. I couldn't stop looking at myself in the mirror. I even attended a party. OMG! It was a miracle. I was healed. It was magical...or so I thought.

Fast forward: Wednesday June 29, 2011, everything flared up again. Within two weeks I was back to square one. And so I went running to see my General Practitioner. Amid much humming and harring as he examined me, he asked me several questions, then said, "Although I'm not a dermatologist, I think that you could possibly have allergies and possibly contact dermatitis. "

Oh crap, I thought. *Here it comes—steroids...again!* And yes, the good doc prescribed prednisone, another steroid.

Prednisone and prednisolone are members of the glucocorticoid class of hormones. Cortisone is an example of a related hormone with which most people are familiar. Glucocorticoid hormones are produced naturally by the adrenal glands, which are located on top of the kidneys, to prepare us for physical exercise and stress. Glucocorticoids influence the immune system to induce anti-inflammatory actions and play a role in the body's feedback system.

Like Mother, Like Daughter

Like mother, like daughter. Did I say that before? Anyhow, this go-round with steroids, I was a teeny weenie bit more non-compliant, a trait I inherited from my Mum. What this actually translates to: I cut the prescribed dose by half. Sure enough, Wow! It was magical. It took care of the problem. Just like that! Or so I thought. Then BAM! In a couple of weeks I was right back to where I started. I was back to square one.

I went to five doctors in all, and they all did and said the same things: a lot of humming and harring and doling out of steroids. I am so my mother's daughter, I didn't even fill the prescriptions.

Epiphany

On 11 August 2011, the day after my 26th wedding anniversary, I had an epiphany. I realized I would have to do something different. I would have to heal myself, because the steroids were taking care of the symptoms and not the cause. I was putting the lid on a pot of boiling water and expecting the flame to go out. I knew, based on my past and professional experience that food truly is *medicine*. And in order to initiate, my body's natural healing response, I would have to cut out all foods known to produce allergies as well as carbohydrates. I explained to my husband that I would be making some dietary changes, which kinda sorta extended to him, by default. So we gave up all obvious sugar, rice, potatoes, pasta, and wheat in all obvious sources.

This worked well, in fact, very well. For several months my skin condition (along with some sinus issues I had) improved by 50%. The only fly in the ointment was that if I chose, which I did semi-frequently, to consume anything outside of my self- imposed diet I had a major flareup.

By early September 2011, I was feeling 100% better. And my skin looked 100% better, also. However, toward the middle of December, my initial euphoria rapidly wore off. I came to the conclusion that, although I was feeling much, much better, "better" wasn't good enough. Any little thing could trigger an episode. I knew I had to take my healing to another level. In fact, I knew what I had to do. I had been this route 31 years ago.

I had to make a commitment to cleansing my body through changing what I was putting into my mouth and the kind of thoughts I was thinking. In regard to thoughts: Your thoughts, my thoughts, the collective thoughts of all of us, become tangible things. The idea or "thought" came to me that I should beef up with veggies, the fruit smoothies I was drinking five days a week. This would create a nutritious drink that would support the cleansing of my body and put me back on a healthy track. I knew I would have to purchase a new blender. I needed something a little more efficient than the one I currently owned.

Thirty-one years ago, I had cleansed and recalibrated my body by eating fresh ripe seasonal fruit, raw vegetables, and lots and lots of green leafy vegetables, along with nuts, seeds and grains. So, I knew this would work. The question was what was I going to do?

Q: Do my thoughts become things?
A: Yes, your thoughts become things. Thoughts are energy that moves into form and out of form and takes the form or shape from your thought process.
Q: By changing my thoughts, can I change my life?
A: Yes! Yes, you can.

But, don't take my word for it. *Do your own due diligence.* Embrace an authentic thought —something you want for yourself, and not what others are dictating you should have. Think about what you want and what it feels like to you to have it. As much as possible, hold on to your thought process of, *what it feels like to you to have it*, no matter what's going on around you. If you are able to do this, watch as *it* manifests from the intangible into tangible form.

CHAPTER 3
INFLUENCES & CHOICES

As I began to seriously reflect on this chapter of my life and health, I started to connect the dots. As the picture emerged, I realized that my thoughts prior to my skin eruptions had been thoughts filled with extreme irritation. I was irritated with people, places and things, but most of all what this picture reflected back to me was the extreme irritation I had with myself. And so, my body, being the obedient vessel that it is, manifested my thoughts and beliefs in a way that I could understand. My skin became hypersensitive and extremely irritated by the things that I was eating.

In fact, this situation—the feelings, the skin eruptions and the steroids—wasn't new to me. I had been this route before. I had even been the body cleanse route, which came after my Near Death Experience, NDE, some 31 years ago. I knew what was going on and I had more than a vague idea as to what I had to do. The tiny, teeny weenie hiccup in this whole thing, was that I just wasn't sure that I wanted to go that route.

From where I was standing, it looked like a lot of sacrificing of a lot of foods that I simply loved. And to be frank, I didn't want to be the sacrificial lamb in my proactive health care. I wanted to be like the average Joe and pop a pill and make it better. Or better yet, think it, and instantly it would be so. I was resentful about giving anything up, even if it meant that I would heal myself.

So, with that thought as a foundation, I kept giving lip service to doing something about my health. I created a façade of staying away from sugars, wheats and starches. And I did stay away from the obvious ones, but in reality, I wasn't doing a damn thing. I wasn't reading labels or researching the food that I was eating. If you know anything about processed and prepackaged foods, you know that they are usually laden with the prerequisite sugar – mainly from corn syrup, wheat, and salt. Although salt wasn't on my hit list it is present in most prepackage foods. Many of them are full of noxious preservatives, all of which, just as an FYI, are truly toxic in accumulative quantities. Then there is the fact that manufacturers are allowed to put things into prepackaged foods and not label the ingredients. This is done legally under the guise to protect their proprietary rights.

Those of you who know me and are getting to know me, know I'm a believer in everyone conducting their *own due diligence*. My challenge to you is, go to the grocery store, and start reading the labels. It doesn't matter what part of the world you live in, you'll garner the same results. You'll see that several of the main ingredients are sugar, whether from fruit, corn, rice, or cane, or chemicals designed to taste like sugar. And then there is salt at astronomical levels, and of course, wheat that is present in the majority of all processed foods. Why wheat, why sugar, why salt? Who on the face of this earth knows why? Especially as research has shown that all the above are proving to be allergens, which over the long haul create chronic illnesses. However, my research coupled with my personal belief tells me *the why* has far more to do with corporate bottom lines than with the short- or long-term concerns for consumer health and health-related issues.

To Vitamix or Not to Vitamix, That's the Question

December rolled into January 2012, which rolled smoothly into February, then without pause into March. All the while, I was pretending to be pep-talking myself into doing something that I really didn't want to do: cleanse my body. In fact, I clearly had no intention of doing anything. I know that because I *wasn't* doing anything, other than giving lip service to getting my health in order. If there is one thing I know about Ms Wendy Lashley Dearborne, it's that if she truly wants to do something, it will take an act of God to stop her.

Take the purchasing of a Vitamix, which I knew would be central to taking control of my health. I had wanted a Vitamix forever, and that would be approximately six or so years forever. I just didn't want to pay for it. And as theft comes with all sorts of negative connotations attached, I felt it best to just keep dreaming and wanting.

I feel sure that for those of you who have purchased a Vitamix and or those of you who are still on the fence, y'all can relate when I screamed, "Four hundred fifty dollars for a bloody blender!? Oh hell NO, I don't think so!"

I am my father's daughter as well as my mother's. Like Dad, I love gadgets. I was absolutely enthralled by the demos that I saw see on a regular basis at Sam's Club or Costco. However, I wasn't quite enslaved enough to get my head around the price tag. So understanding my dilemma, my girl friend Tracy K gave me $200 as a birthday gift in February and told me it was going toward "Wendy's Vitamix fund."

On April 18th, while I was shopping in Costco, the Vitamix crew were giving demonstrations. After I had had my fill of smoothies, soup, and ice cream, all made with this amazing machine, I asked the presenter how long they would be in Costco. He said that they would be leaving next week, on Thursday. In my jazzy, upbeat way, I told him I would be back next Wednesday to purchase my Vitamix. He gave me a very bored look that said, "Whatever lady! I've heard that a million times." As you read this, I know you are asking, "Why didn't you purchase it then?" The answer is simple. I still had to get my head around it. "It" being the price tag of four hundred and fifty dollars.

In between April 18th and Wednesday April 25th, I happened to watch a documentary called *Fat Sick & Nearly Dead*. You can stream this from Netflix or Amazon Prime. I watch lots of documentaries as part of the research I do for *My Life My Choice!*, the internet radio show that I produce and host. I have seen most of the documentaries available on the state of the food industry and how our lives are being impacted. Ironically, *Fat Sick & Nearly Dead* had been in my queue for ages and I just kept bypassing it. As my Mum always says, "Nothing before its time." And my time had definitely come.

I urge you to watch it. The information presented in this reality documentary transformed my life in amazing ways, and it's only begun to scratch the surface, because new things are being revealed to me daily.

How did watching this documentary transform my life? What I mean by this is that watching *Fat Sick & Nearly Dead* allowed me to make choices regarding my health and life. It encouraged me to take control by being proactive about my own health. And it gave me in a generalized way the tools to do it.

The premise of the movie is this: An Australian and an American meet up at a truck stop in middle America. Both have a rare skin condition that is only treatable through traditional medicine by taking steroids orally. They were each told that this is as good as it gets. They were both told that taking steroids is what they have to do for the rest of their lives. The maker of the movie made the choice to do something different. He decided to use food, namely, the juice of green, live, organic foods as medicine to cure himself! And juicing worked for him, so well that he was cured. And it also worked for the guy he met at the truck stop.

Needless to say, all sorts of bells and whistles went off inside my head as I watched this documentary. They had a skin condition that could only be treated/controlled by steroids. I had a skin condition that had been treated by steroids, which only served to cover the underlying issue. And I also had a skin condition that was responding favorably to a change in diet, as did theirs. In short, I identified with the lead characters. I felt their pain as if it were my own.

A Stranger's Influence

You never know who, what, or where your life-changing insights will come from. As I lay in bed reflecting on everything that I had just watched, my mind set up two camps: the "Buy the Vitamix!" camp and the "Really Wendy? Four hundred fifty dollars for a blender? I don't think so!" camp vying for my attention. After a considerable amount of time spent going back and forth between the two camps and getting nowhere, I decided to surrender and allow the Universe to support me in my decision making process by giving me a definite sign.

As this is a process that I use often, I was on alert for a sign or directive. The next morning, bright and early, out of the blue my message came. I spoke with my friend and fellow coach Lois Johnson. She was so excited, because she had received from her Aunt Tommie's estate a high-speed blender and had been making fruit and vegetable smoothies and juices. Lois talked enthusiastically about her blender and some of the creations she had made. She spoke about how fantastic she was feeling and how her energy levels were up. She was inspired to grow her own organic, green leafy vegetables in a community gardening program here in Las Vegas.

As we spoke about her juicing and the positive ways in which her life had been impacted, I was struck by the fact that I hadn't had an opportunity to meet Lois's aunt. And yet, indirectly she had given me the message to go ahead and purchase my Vitamix. The knock-on effect of being influenced by this stranger is that I am now sharing *Green Is 4 Life: A Simple Guide To Creating Life-Giving Green Smoothies* with you.

The next day, Wednesday April 25, I went back to Costco and purchased my Vitamix. Thank you Aunt Tommie! Thank you, too Tracy K, for starting "Wendy's Vitamix Fund." One friend and one stranger, you both have helped me transform my life!

Six weeks later, on June 16, 2012, I began what turned into a 35-day green smoothie fast, to recalibrate my metabolism and boost my immune system, using food as medicine to heal myself. It was a resounding success. In the next chapters, you will explore the foundation of creating your Green Is 4 Life smoothies. You will also become familiar with the nuts and bolts of what is required to make and integrate delicious and nutritious green smoothies into your life.

Q: Do I need to know what and when things went wrong in my life to make changes?
A: While it is helpful to know the origin, it is much more helpful to know what you want and where you want to go. You can then create a plan to get there.
Q: Do we get signs and signals along the way to help us?
A: Yes! That is your intuition doing what it does best…providing you with insights from unknown sources so that you can make an informed choice.

CHAPTER 4
WHAT IS A GREEN SMOOTHIE?

Using Food as Medicine

A green smoothie is a delicious, naturally creamy concoction of luscious naturally ripened fruits, crisp garden vegetables, and tender leafy greens that have been pulverized into a liquid by a blender, preferably a high-speed blender like a Vitamix. It is a simple way of taking in large quantities of raw vegetables combined with fruits in a palatable way. It's a deliberate way of selecting raw foods for their healing properties and their nutritional benefits. It's ultimately about choosing to use food as medicine.

Fresh foods in their natural state—fruits, vegetables and herbs, even organically grown meat and wild-caught fish—have been created by nature to provide everything that you need to keep you healthy in mind, body and spirit. Chemically laden, processed foods have been created by man to fill an emotional need in your life. Example: Fast and prepackaged foods. No real planning, shopping, or preparation is required on your part. This gives the illusion of freeing up your time. It's one less thing for you to cram into your already overextended day. But in the long run at the cost of your health, is it really worth it?

Also, you never hear, (or at least I've never heard this) "OMG! You've been dumped! Let me grab the fruit salad and two spoons. Or let me grab the veggie tray and spinach and eggplant dip and I'll be right over." No, what you'll hear is, "Let me grab the ice-cream (or cheese cake or mac and cheese) and two spoons. Girlfriend, I'm on my way!" It's my belief that processed foods are geared psychologically to support our emotional deficits and not to bring nutritional value or balance to the whole: the mind, body, and spirit.

What Makes A Smoothie?

My yummy young coconut water, hazelnut, sun-kissed black cherries, sweet carrots, crisp celery, luscious ripe bananas and one bunch of dark green curly kale with a hit of fragrant peppermint smoothie has come under much scrutiny. The above recipe taste like chocolate...to me...and has been called some very unflattering names, from sludge to mud, and a few choice words in between, which can't be printed.

I've witness my clients shiver ever so delicately and prettily wrinkle their noses. And then others shudder not so delicately, curling their lips and turning up their noses. And then we have the "hurl crew" namely TCK, RR, ALP, SJB (You know who you are). They literally look like they want to hurl at the thought of drinking this concoction. However, with all that, they are curious enough about my transformation to ask "So, if and only if, I decide to drink that stuff, what can I put in it?" People have even asked, "Can I have a sip?" or, "So what's in this one this time?"

Your green smoothie is broken down into four segments:

➢ Fluids
➢ Vegetables
➢ Greens
➢ Fruit

Why Fluids?

Many fruits, vegetables, and green leafy veggies have a high water content, but it's not high enough to create a drinkable smoothie. When fruits and veggies are put into a high-speed blender without water or nut milk, you will create a puree, even when using citrus or melons. This is because the cellulose and fibrous parts of the plants are included and not excluded, as they are when juicing, from the blend. And as a result of the inclusion of fiber, your smoothie will need either nature's universal solvent, water, or nut milks. Your green smoothie requires fluid to assist in pulverizing your fruits, nuts, vegetables and green leafy veggies to just the right consistency.

Note that the correct consistency is subject to personal choice. Some like their smoothies to be thick, like an old-fashioned malt shake, while others like their smoothies to be the consistency of half-and-half. Without fluid, whether it's coconut water, water, or nut milk your smoothie may end up the consistency of baby food, too thick to drink through a straw, yet not thick enough to eat with a fork. In other words, you will wind up with a vegetable/fruit puree. This can work too, if this is your choice, but most of us prefer something drinkable.

Water also allows you to experiment with various milks—almond, coconut, cashew (my personal favorite), Brazil nut, hazelnut (another favorite), pecan, etc. You name the nut and you can create milk with it, this includes peanuts, which happen to be my least favorite of all nuts. Then there are the milks made from grains, seeds, and berries—oat, hemp, sesame, barley, rice, soy, and the list goes on—all of which require water for their creation.

Why Vegetables?

In addition to having their own natural, unique sweetness, vegetables, much like fruits, bring fiber, trace minerals, water, and other life-giving properties to your green smoothie equation. They also create a solid foundational latticework, which is designed to support the healthy detoxification and cleansing of cells within the body, through the exchange of cellular fluids.

Vegetables are also instrumental in helping you to create the right consistency for your smoothie. They add the earthy element of depth, tone, texture and of course color. Because there is such an abundant array of seasonal veggies available, the chance of becoming bored is slim to none.

Why Green Leafy Vegetables?

In two words, "liquid sunshine!" In addition to the fiber, water, trace minerals, and vitamins, greens provide chlorophyll, which in some circles is known as liquid sunshine. Chlorophyll is in the plant world is what blood is to us humans. Both are chemically similar in composition with just one difference, chlorophyll being centered around the element magnesium, while blood is centered on the element iron.

Chlorophyll is the green pigment in plants, which supports metabolic functions such as respiration, elimination, and growth. Chlorophyll absorbs energy from the sun to facilitate photosynthesis.

Research has indicated that the ingestion of chlorophyll has excellent health benefits for humans.

Health Benefits of Chlorophyll

The chlorophyll present in green leafy vegetables has been shown to provide some amazing health benefits through its anti-oxidant, anti-inflammatory, and wound-healing properties.

It supports the growth and repair of tissue.
It oxygenates the blood.
It neutralizes free radicals.
It supports healthy elimination.
It supports healthy respiration.
It encourages the growth of beneficial intestinal flora.
It promotes the assimilation of food.
It boosts and supports the immune system.
It reduces inflammation.

Chlorophyll has been shown to do this and much, much more. Again, I'm all about you conducting *your own due diligence*. Be your own cold hard fact!

Why Fruit?

Fruits are optional in your smoothie. However, they are an important option to be considered as they bring several significant aspects to your green smoothie equation. First and foremost, fruits give you the ability to customize your smoothie to suit your taste buds. They enhance and complement the taste of all vegetables. And if some greens are too strong-tasting for you, fruits can be used to moderate their taste.

Some of the more popular greens used in smoothies, like kale, chard or tender spinach, when blended in large quantities can taste bitter, thus making your smoothie unpalatable. Fruits, luscious and ripe, give natural sweetness to your blend, eliminating the need to use processed sweeteners, artificial or otherwise. In addition to being delicious, ripe fruits deliver vitamins, minerals, micronutrients, water, fiber, texture, and thickness, which all support you in creating the perfect "Green Is 4 Life" smoothie.

Color Matters

Another consideration in the creation of your green smoothie is the color of both your fruits and vegetables. Where would you be without color in your life? I want you to take a moment to think about your favorite colors and the impact they have on your life. Do they make you feel powerful, serene, courageous, sexy, happy, contented, tranquil, safe and secure, or hungry? Is your favorite color hot, cold, warm, cool, and tingly? Is it wet or dry? Is it silent, like a whisper, or loud, like thunder?

Color is a living, vibrating thing and is a powerful, influential force in our lives, but one often overlooked and often understated. Color can be used *consciously*, as a viable tool to help us to create the lives we want to live. Color can help us achieve better health, more wealth, and improved relationships with others and self, along with spiritual and creative expression and development.

When you think about the color of fruits and vegetables, even nuts, they are just like an artist's palette. When combined together and ingested they have the ability to affect us in numerous subtle ways. Color heals; color encourages; color motivates. It empowers; it energizes; it influences your moods, and it connects you to all people and all things in the earthly and heavenly realms.

The vibrant color of fruits and vegetables is something worth exploring. *New Chakra Healing* by Cyndi Dale and *Color Book* by Lori Reid can give you greater insight into the role color plays in your life and how to use it.

Using the four foundational segments that green smoothies are created from, you can begin to see that there are endless combinations that you can make as you create your Green Is 4 Life smoothie.

Q: Why do I require fluid in my smoothies?
A: Apart from helping to stay hydrated, fluids (in the form of coconut water, water, and nut, seed and grain milks) allow you

to customize and boost your smoothies, by integrating the natural nutritional elements that they bring.

CHAPTER 5
WHAT'S IN IT FOR ME?

As I thought about this question, "What's in it for me?" my mind automatically went to the payoff and reward system that we all live by: what we are prepared to give, the payoff, to get what we want, the reward. As humans, we are goal-orientated creatures. This is part of the intrinsic human condition. We must have something to work towards that we feel will be beneficial or good for us. Otherwise we won't do it. We work toward the reward by doing things that will get us there.

So what's in this for you? What benefit will you derive from adding green smoothies to your life? I can only talk about my personal experience and the experiences of my clientele who have included green smoothies into their diets.

In my case, as you read earlier it was all about taking control of my health in a way that was proactive and not detrimental to me physiologically, psychologically, emotionally, and spiritually. The principal benefit was eliminating the underlying cause of the chronic skin condition that had plagued me for several years.

That was my goal: to eliminate what was causing my skin to crack open and bleed. I have enough healing knowledge to know that the skin disorder was just a symptom, alerting me to look for an underlying cause. So my goal was to get to the cause.

Just like all the doctors I went to see, I didn't know what the cause of my problem was. However, with my training as a holistic practitioner, I did know that most diseases and disorders arise from a depressed immune system, with origins that stem from diet, emotions, and immobility. I decided to start by boosting my immune system and in the process cleansing my blood and body. Green smoothies were new to me; however, the concept of plant-based healing was one I had some experience of, 31 years ago, with a book called *Back to Eden* written by Jethro Kloss.

After watching *Fat Sick & Nearly Dead* and buying my Vitamix—thanks Tracy!—I elected to go on a 35-day green smoothie fast. IT CHANGED MY LIFE! Those 35 days changed my life in ways that I hadn't even anticipated.

One of the major benefits that most people experience is a surge of energy, along with increased feelings of vitality. Many report a reduction in sinus and allergy complaints and better sleep. If you suffer from chronic sinusitis and allergies or insomnia and are currently taking any of the OTC medications, adding green smoothies to your diet might be something worth looking at.

Besides the above-mentioned, other benefits can be, but are not limited to, the following:

- ✓ Improved vision
- ✓ Lessened cravings for carbs and sugar
- ✓ Cessation of nicotine cravings
- ✓ Healthy glowing skin
- ✓ Arrested bleeding of gums
- ✓ Regulation of bowel movements
- ✓ Expelling of mucus
- ✓ Deeper meditations
- ✓ Clarity of mind
- ✓ Clean tongue
- ✓ Balancing of metabolism
- ✓ Tranquility, calmness
- ✓ Shiny hair
- ✓ Stronger nails
- ✓ The ability to stop eating when full
- ✓ Lack of desire for processed foods
- ✓ Healing faster without scarring

✓ Dissolving of scarred tissue
✓ Anti-inflammatory action on joints
✓ Reduction of aches and pains
✓ Toning and cleansing of liver
✓ Cleansing and toning of digestive tract
✓ Better digestion and nutrient and micronutrient assimilation
✓ Cleansing of blood and kidneys
✓ Efficient cell rejuvenation
✓ Lessened mood swings and a more balanced temperament
✓ Reduction of hot flashes and night sweats
✓ Increased muscle tone
✓ More flexibility
✓ Elimination of gas and bloating
✓ Loss of desire to eat meat
✓ Permanent weight loss

Yeah, you can experience all this and more by adding green smoothies to your diet. And you can kick-start much of the above by going on a green smoothie fast. The fantastic thing about green smoothies is that you don't have to fast for 60, 30, 20, or even 10 days to derive some of the benefits listed above. Three days is ample.

Why Would I Do This?

This question has been posed to me time and time again, by family, friends, clients, and radio show listeners. "Wendy, why would I want to do this? Why would I want to give up food, and drink smoothies?"

My answer is simple: "How could you not exhaust all options to get you to optimal health?" I say this not because it worked for me and thousands of others like me, but because adding green smoothies to your diet is another option. It provides you with another choice, and remember this: Life—my life, your life, our life—is built one choice at a time.

I won't tell you that you must add green smoothies to your diet or even go as far as suggesting that you go on a green smoothie fast. What I will do is present my facts, and please note, I said *my facts*, which are based on my own experiences and those of my clientele. I will tell you to be your own cold, hard statistic, by suggesting that you *do your own due diligence* and letting your experience with green smoothies speak for itself. In short, why should you do this? Because you have nothing to lose and everything to gain! That's why!

Q: Will I benefit from drinking a smoothie daily?
A: Yes. Drinking a smoothie daily can and will provide you with fresh fruits and vegetables and their nutrients—protein, vitamins, fiber and minerals.

CHAPTER 6
WEIGHT LOSS

Will you experience weight loss drinking green smoothies and or going on a green smoothie fast?

The answer to that question is yes. However, *Green Is 4 Life* isn't a book about weight loss. It's all about changing your current dietary lifestyle with the inclusion of raw, live, life-giving fruits, nuts, grains, seeds, vegetables and green leafy vegetables.

Weight loss is a definite side effect when conducting a green smoothie fast. And some people have reported weight loss as a result of incorporating green smoothies into their current dietary regime.

Please understand that any time you restrict or exclude something that you have eaten on a regular basis from your diet, you will experience weight loss. By eliminating all obvious sugars, wheat (Yes, that included bread, cakes, cookies.), and processed foods and beefing up his intake of raw fresh vegetables, Dee, my husband shed more than 50 pounds. He was only drinking the occasional green smoothie and eating lots of salads…green leafy vegetables, lots of vegetables and plenty of seasonal ripe fruit. He was following the Dietary Principle. (See chapter 7.)

While some do lose weight, and you will find reams of information on the internet about green smoothies and dieting, I don't advocate using this method as a quick fix for unwanted pounds. I advocate adding green smoothies into your diet as a choice for a healthier lifestyle.

You may be asking the question "have you lost weight Wendy?" No, I haven't lost weight. I've shed unwanted toxicity in the form of pounds and in the process, I've shed three dress sizes. What I still find amazing some seven months later is that I've also shed the desire or craving to eat sugar, carbs, and red meat. I'm now a pescetarian, which means I eat shellfish and seafood.

CHAPTER 7
THE DIETARY PRINCIPLE

If there is one thing that I would like you to take away with you from reading this book it would be *the Dietary Principle*. Why? Because it has the power to change your life forever should you choose to adopt it.

There is a saying, "You are what you eat," and there is much truth in that. It doesn't make it bad or good. It just IS. I know that I have written this book primarily about the inclusion of raw, life-giving foods into your current dietary lifestyle, in the form of a green smoothie. However, it's important to note that whether your vegetables are uncooked, steamed, stir-fried, roasted, sautéed, or just simply boiled this life-changing Dietary Principle applies to everyone. It is for vegans, vegetarians, pescetarians, and flexitarians.

Let me stop for some brief definitions here. A vegan eats no animal products—no milk or eggs—and no meat of any kind. A vegetarian or ovo-lacto-vegetarian usually eats milk products and eggs, but no meat. A pescetarian eats fish and shellfish, but no other meat. A flexitarian eats meat, fish and dairy produces only occasionally.

Whether you don't eat meat or any animal products, just eat fish, or eat everything, applying this principle to your life can dramatically change how you look, how you think, and how you feel about yourself.

The Dietary Principle is simple and easy to follow and can be integrated into any dietary lifestyle anywhere in the world. The universal format in which nature grows a plant is the same here, there, or wherever you happen to be.

The Dietary Principle was given to me by a very wise man almost 30 years ago. It has been the gift that keeps on giving, because it has changed my life and that of others and will continue to do so.

Kofi was a close friend of my late sister Rosemarie Jennifer, who had come to say his goodbyes and to console us during her untimely passing.

As we sat and talked about life and death, he told me that when you sit down to eat, the food on your plate (or as in your case now, the green smoothie in your glass) should reflect the growth cycle of a plant. I didn't understand what he meant. "Reflect the growth cycle of a plant?" He went on to explain that when you sit down to eat, present on your plate should be foods from the root through to the life-giving seed.

When I first heard this concept, something stirred deep within me, and a spiritual tsunami took place. That paradigm shift had me in awe and it still does. And as I look back on my cooking and eating style, I can see clearly, that subconsciously I have, to varying degrees, applied this principle for the last 29 years. Little did I know at the time, the impact that our conversation filled with words of wisdom, would come to have on my life and the lives of others I have touched.

So what does this really mean? On your plate or in your Mason jar, you have the parts of a plant. You should always have part:

Of the root
Of the stem
Of the leaf
Of the fruit
Of the seed

All the above represents a whole plant. If you think about a full-grown tree, you'll note that it has roots. It has a trunk, branches and twigs, along with leaves and it usually bears some kind of fruit that will produce a seed – a seed from where it originated and can reproduce itself. When you look at any mature, fruit-bearing plant, like corn, carrots, rice etc. you are witnessing the Universal Alpha and Omega of life. The beginning and end of the plant...the cycle begins with the seed and ends with the seed.

Let's take a look at this concept in a little more detail.

Root vegetables. They are the starchy or earthy type of vegetables that grow underground. Carrots, parsnips, turnips, beets, potatoes, to name but a few, fall into this category.

The stem of a plant in this instance refers to the part of the plant that is between the root and the leaves. The stems tend to be a little more fibrous in texture. Leeks, green onions, broccoli, celery, cauliflower etc.

The leaf of a plant is located at the top end of the stem and between it and the fruit/flower. Spinach, kale, chard, beets, collards, mustard and dandelion greens, etc.

The fruit is whatever the plant bears. Peaches, pears, oranges, green peppers, green onions, garlic, cucumber, potatoes, cauliflower, beets, cherries, etc.

The seed is inside the fruit and is anything that will grow and reproduce itself. Beans, legumes, rice, corn, wheat, nuts, etc.

Herbs are leaves, and spices are mostly seeds. They are used for their flavor or medicinal properties and are optional.

The above-mentioned only scratches the surface. And you can see where you can start building your green smoothie or your dinner plate with ease. One of my favorite smoothies is made with carrots (root), celery (stem), chard (leaf), cherries (fruit), and cashew nuts (seed), with a hint of peppermint and coconut water.

What Should Be In My Smoothie?

➤ Root vegetables
➤ Stems of vegetables
➤ Green leafy vegetables
➤ Fruits or anything that the plant bears
➤ Seeds, nuts and grains. These can be added in the form of milks. (See chapter 19 on how to make your own nut milks.)

Herbs and spices are a fantastic way of supporting the digestive system and adding micronutrients to your green smoothie equation. They also infuse a touch of *je ne sais quoi,* bringing out your own unique expression. Herbs are optional and should be used sparingly, as they have the ability to overpower your smoothie and make it unpalatable.

Meat Eaters & The Dietary Principle

For pescetarians, flexitarians, and meat-eaters in general, we add categories to the Dietary Principle. We eat

Of the root
Of the stem
Of the leaf
Of the fruit
Of the seed
Of the sea: fish and shellfish
Of the land: meat and the products of animals, like cheese, milk, etc.
Of the air: poultry and eggs

What should your plate look like? The food on your plate should look like a beautiful, vibrant, healthy plant! Whether your veggies are cooked or uncooked, two-thirds or more of the food on your plate should be devoted to vegetables. One-third can be divided between the sea, land or air. FYI: So as not to overtax the digestive system and aid in assimilation and optimal absorption, it is best to eat only one type of animal, whether fish, meat, or poultry, in one sitting.

Q: Does my green smoothie have to contain an entire plant for it to be beneficial?
A: No. You can obtain much benefit without your smoothie's containing an entire plant.

Choosing to create your green life-giving smoothie using the Dietary Principle takes it to another level. Just like using the color of fruits and vegetables and the nutritional enhancement found in coconut water, nuts, seeds and grains will boost the healing potential of your smoothie.

CHAPTER 8
THE POWER OF WATER

There are many things that we can live without, but water isn't one of them. Water is the foundation of everything. Water sustains life as we know it and the lack of it spells certain disaster.

We often understate the important and integral role of water in our lives. The very fact that it's so vital makes us take it for granted, even when it's in short supply. Perhaps a better word would be complacent; we are complacent about it. Again, until we don't have it—then and only then, do we realize how much we depend on it and need it.

Water, as we have tragically seen over the past few years has the ability to wreak havoc, washing away entire areas leaving nothing behind. It can wear away diamond, the hardest substance known to man, and, yet, has the ability to nurture, protect, and feed an unborn child. Water is our everything and rightly so, considering that the human body is comprised of 75% to 85% water.

Water plays and integral part in the creation of your green smoothies and the inclusion of green smoothies in your life, particularly if you decide on doing a green smoothie fast.

There are numerous theories, studies and statistics circulating about water and how much water you should be drinking. Eight glasses per day? Two gallons per day? Half your body weight in fluid ounces? Then there is the type of water: reverse osmosis filtered water, oxygenated with O2 drops, alkaline, acidic, bottled, tap water, filtered, unfiltered, cold or hot, still or carbonated? Whatever theory you subscribe to, the one thing that they all have in common, is that water and the drinking of it are essential to maintaining life and health.

Intake of fluids into the body assists in maintaining the metabolic functions that are essential for life. Water aids in detoxification, elimination, assimilation, and absorption processes. It assists in the cleansing of the cells and the healing of the body. As I'm fond of saying, this is only the "nano-tip" of the iceberg. So yes, the power of water is needed for you to create your perfect Green Is 4 Life smoothie.

Before we explore the role water plays in the creation of your green smoothies, I want to share a fact that Coach Olivia Lashley and My Life My choice radio show co-host unearthed. This fact left me speechless! *Nothing burns without water present.*

Coach Olivia came across this little fact while conducting research into water and its powerful abilities for a show that we aired last year. *Nothing burns without water present,* hammered home the point that water is one of the most important substances known to man. You don't think of kindling as having water, but for the kindling to burn, even though it appears dry to us, there is water present. Amazing!

Do I Need Water For My Green Smoothie?

Yes, you do…or at least you need some sort of fluid, which as I mention earlier, will contain a large percentage of water. This is irrespective of whether it is pure water, coconut water, or water that is present in nut milks. Water is used in the creation of your green smoothie to assist in the blending process. This is an important step as it turns your fruit and vegetable from a lumpy, slushy puree to a full-bodied, smooth, creamy-textured drink.

Coconut water

Coconut water from young coconuts is considered to be a super food and is packed full of naturally occurring nutrients, vitamins, minerals and trace minerals, all of which are needed to sustain life in a healthy way. Coconut water can give your green smoothie a natural turbo-boost that takes your nutritional drink to another level.

Coconut water from young coconuts is purported to have more potassium than bananas and in some cases more vitamins than fruits. Another benefit of coconut water is its antiviral, antiparasitic, antimicrobial and antibacterial properties. Coconut water is given to people in the tropics when they have digestive disruptions like gastric flue, constipation, or diarrhea. It is given to hydrate and replenish the body with life-giving nutrients.

Coconut water has the ability to rehydrate the body and is nature's answer to Gatorade. It is a rich source of electrolytes, thereby supporting your body's ability to send and receive uninterrupted electrical impulses. Coconut water can influence the healthy function of your heart and cells. The nutritional value of the water from the young coconut makes it worthy of serious consideration as a staple in your pantry. It is also an excellent choice as the base for making your own nut, seed, grain milks and for your green smoothies.

Q: Do I have to drink eight glasses of water a day?
A: No, not eight glasses, but I do advocate while conducting a green smoothie fast that you always start your day out with 32 ounces of room-temperature spring water, optionally, with a twist of lemon. I do suggest that you drink at least two glasses of pure water per day when including smoothies in your current dietary practice.
Q: How much coconut water can I drink per day?
A: I suggest no more than 16 – 24 fluid ounces, as it can act as a very mild laxative.
Q: If I've been ill with diarrhea and vomiting, can I drink coconut water?
A: It will be one of the best things that you can drink to rehydrate your body, and because of the antibacterial action, and it can assist in bringing the digestive ecology back into balance.
Q: Can coconut water hydrate me?
A: Yes much like Gatorade, coconut water can encourage your body to absorb the water it needs.

CHAPTER 9
ORGANIC VS. NON-ORGANIC

The word "organic" refers to the way certain farmers grow and process agricultural products, which include fruits, vegetables, grains, nuts, dairy products, fish, and meat. Once upon a time, you could only find organic produce in health-food stores or by becoming a member of a community farming co-operative. Now organic food sits side by side next to conventionally grown food. Other than the barcode, which begins with the number 9, it can be difficult to tell them apart.

Organic farmers don't use conventional methods to fertilize, control weeds, or prevent or treat livestock diseases. Organic farmers conduct more-sophisticated crop rotations and spread mulch or manure to keep weeds at bay, as opposed to using chemical weed killers.

Organic	Non-organic
Use natural fertilizers, such as manure or compost, to feed soil and plants.	Use chemical fertilizers to promote plant growth and artificially replenish the soil.

Spray pesticides from natural sources; use beneficial insects and birds, mating disruption, or traps to reduce pests and disease.	Spray synthetic insecticides to reduce pests and disease.
Use environmentally-generated plant-killing compounds; rotate crops, till, hand weed, or mulch to manage weeds.	Use synthetic herbicides to manage weeds.
Give animals organic feed and allow them to graze outdoors and reach natural maturity. Use rotational grazing, a balanced diet and clean housing to help minimize disease.	Administer antibiotics, growth hormones and medications to prevent disease and spur growth.

There is a raging debate as to whether organic food is better for you than conventional food. Before I give my very personal and professional opinion, I will once again make the suggestion that you *do your own due diligence*. Allow your experience, your taste buds, to give you the information that you need to make an informed decision about the produce you buy that will ultimately affect you and your family.

When it comes to organic and non-organic, my experience has shown me that there is a huge difference in the taste, smell, texture, and mouthfeel of organic produce, fish and meat. It even cooks differently. When my taste buds experience the vitality of organic fruits and vegetables, you will hear me say, "Wow! This reminds me of when I was a child. I haven't tasted an apple like this in years."

However, you will pay dearly for that "Wow" taste. Organic produce is expensive and sometimes in my opinion, a little over-priced. Another factor to consider is that the shelf life of organic produce often appears to be much shorter than that of conventionally grown and raised produce.

That being said, life is about choices and for the most part, I choose organic. If you are interested in learning more about organic food and its impact on your health, the environment, and of course your wallet, check out *What to Eat: Food That's Good for Your Health, Pocket and Plate* by Joanna Blythman. Also, this book is a must: *Food Rules: An Eater's Manual* by Michael Pollan. This wonderful book simplifies the rules for eating and shopping.

So Do I Use Organic or Non-Organic Produce in My Green Smoothies?

The answer to that question is simple: Start where you are at. Buying all organic fruits and vegetables can be costly. If you are on a fixed budget, it can and will break the bank. The knock-on effect from that is that you may decide you can't afford to add green smoothies into your life. That would be a pity. Once again, start where you are at.

If your current budget is for conventionally-grown produce, start there. Add in the occasional organic fruit or vegetable and conduct your own comparison check. Do your own due diligence. Does it taste any different? Is it sweeter, sharper, more pungent or bitter, etc.? Does it improve the texture of your green smoothie and do you notice any difference in your digestion?

Much of the information that you will find online will tell you that if you aren't going to use or invest in using organic produce when making your smoothies, then there's no point in doing a cleanse or changing your diet. I disagree, strongly. Even if you are conducting a green smoothie fast to cleanse your body, as I did for 35 days, I advise you to *start where you are at*. Use conventionally grown produce if that is where you are at, organic if that is where you are at, or a mixture of both. The most important thing is to start.

A suggestion for adding organic produce to your diet is to look into some options beyond the supermarket—like your local farming community. Another option to think about is growing your own produce in a local community farming project, or better yet, start one of your own. And of course, you can sign up and join a co-operative that delivers a weekly organic basket. You'll find if you split this between two or more people, it is a very economical and cost effective way of buying fresh organic produce.

Just as an FYI: I use both. I'm predominately organic, however I do use conventionally grown produce.

Q: Do I have to use all organic produce in my green smoothie?
A: No. However, it's preferable.
Q: If I don't use organic produce in my green smoothie will I get any health benefits?
A: Yes! Yes! And Yes! You will be able to derive many, many health-giving benefits from your smoothie.

Start where you are at! Organic or non-organic. The important thing is that you START.

PART TWO

CHAPTER 10
GREEN SMOOTHIE FASTING

"Humans live on one-quarter of what they eat; on the other three-quarters lives their doctor." ~ Egyptian pyramid inscription, 3800 B.C.

Let's take a look at green smoothie fasting. As I stated in an earlier chapter, I completed a 35-day green smoothie fast to take care of the underlying issues that were causing the systemic skin problem I had. I used green smoothies to recalibrate my metabolism and boost my very, very underactive and compromised immune system. And I was successful. Very successful! The problem and symptoms where eradicated.

Green Smoothie vs. Juicing

I elected to carry out a green smoothie fast as opposed to a juice fast, because I couldn't get my head around discarding all the pulp that was left after pressing the juice out of the fruits and vegetables. It seemed like such a big waste of nutrients, a huge waste of produce and, of course, a huge waste of money. And in addition to that, if using a centrifuge juicer, the fruits for juicing were limited to apples and pears.

Softer fruits like peaches, plums, persimmons, nectarines, mangos, papaya, melons, strawberries, bananas and avocado to name but a few where all ruled out of the process. Not to mention making your own nut and grain milks.

After watching the movie *Fat Sick & Nearly Dead*, I started my fast by creating green smoothies using my Vitamix and straining them in a nut milk bag to get the juice. A nut milk bag is a large drawstring pouch made of nylon, hemp or cheesecloth and used to strain the pulp from seed, nut or grain milks. I kept this up for four days. As I lay in bed that Thursday night, I knew intrinsically that I wouldn't be able to go the 30-day distance juicing. This was because it was just plain wrong having all that good stuff, life-giving fiber, go to waste.

As I lay there allowing my mind to roam, I was suddenly struck by a thought. Well, it was more than a thought. It was my intuition giving me a strong directive to get up NOW and look up green smoothie fasting. For a while, I just lay there thinking, *Oh for goodness sakes. This is ridiculous, it's two minutes past midnight.* On the heels of that thought, my intuition kicked in again telling me to get up NOW and look online. Reluctantly…okay huffily, very huffily…I did just that. I went into my office, woke my PC up, and typed "green smoothie fasting" into the search box. Poof! Just like that, I was inundated with information that I used to transform my life.

So What Is Green Smoothie Fasting?

Fasting, in my usage, is when you willingly abstain from doing something that you normally do. This can be abstinence from any activity, from watching the news to eating chocolate. Fasting can be mental, physical, and/or emotional abstinence.

Health professionals of most cultures throughout history have recommended fasting as therapy for various conditions. What they found, and continue to be fascinated by, is that fasting initiates the body's own healing response. It has been shown to improve many ailments.

And so it is with green smoothie fasting. *Green Is 4 Life* is all about your abstaining from eating certain foods and drinks for a period of time. By doing this, you free energy, initiating your intrinsic healing response. When you stop and think about all the food you eat, some good, but much of it highly processed or not so good, you can begin to see why you maybe a little or a lot off-kilter. How this imbalance presents itself is in the manifestation of some disease or disorder. This can be mental, physical, or emotional/spiritual. When fasting from eating certain foods, physiological, psychological, and emotional/spiritual recalibration takes place. Green smoothie fasting will

➢ Rest the digestive system
➢ Improve assimilation and digestion of food
➢ Curb cravings
➢ Allow for cleansing and detoxification of the body
➢ Cleanse the blood
➢ Boost immune system
➢ Support lymphatic function
➢ Create a break in eating patterns and help identify problems
➢ Promote greater mental clarity and dexterity
➢ Heal "stuck" emotional patterns
➢ Increase feelings of physical strength,
➢ Increasing energy levels
➢ Promote an inner stillness, enhancing spiritual connection
➢ Promote calm
➢ Increase self-awareness
➢ Reduce edema
➢ Clear skin
➢ Promote healthy sleep patterns
➢ Reduce stress
➢ Encourage healthy and speedy cell regeneration
➢ Improve the five senses
➢ Deepen meditation and spiritual connections

Reaching into all areas of your life, these benefits and more are what you can and will experience when green smoothie fasting.

Q: Are juicing and smoothies the same thing?
A: Smoothies include all the plant pulp and fiber. Juicing discards this pulp and fiber.
Q: Do I need fiber in my diet?
A: Yes. Fiber supports your metabolic functions and increases the efficiency of your intestinal tract. Fiber is also instrumental in the body's absorption of water.

Q: Can I juice and derive all the health benefits listed above?
A: Yes.

CHAPTER 11
HOW LONG TO FAST FOR

The experience of fasting begins with your making a conscious choice. You can start out simply with a short-term fast, or go for an intermediate or long-term fast, which is more complex. The choice is yours.

Short fast	1 – 3 days.
Intermediate fast	4 - 7 days.
Long term fast	8 days or more.

Whether you choose one day or, as in my case, 35 days, you will derive much benefit from fasting. And the results of fasting touch all areas of your life.

Fasting also gives your body, digestive tract, and organs a much needed chance to rest, repair and heal. It also allows you to begin the process of reconnecting to your physical, emotional, and spiritual self. As with all things that have the potential to impact your body and mind, check with your medical health care professional before going on a green smoothie fast.

Preparing For Your Fast

There are several key things to consider when undertaking a green smoothie fast. These elements are the foundation for your success.

> ➤ Why have you chosen to conduct a green smoothie fast?
> ➤ What is your current state of health?
> ➤ Are you healthy enough to participate in a green smoothie fast?
> ➤ Do you require medical supervision while conducting your green smoothie fast?
> ➤ How long do you want to fast for?
> ➤ One to three days, four to seven days, or eight days or more?
> ➤ Is the timing right?
> ➤ Do you have commitments that will influence the success of your desired outcome?
> ➤ Will you be working throughout your fast?
> ➤ Do you have all the equipment to make the process easier?
> ➤ How are you going to transport and store your green smoothie and keep it cool?
> ➤ Have you decided on organic, non-organic, or a combination of both kinds of produce?
> ➤ What sweetener, if any, are you going to use?
> ➤ Will you let family, friends, and colleagues know what you are doing? Or will you have a prepared answer that prevents them from probing or trying to force feed you?
> ➤ Do you understand the general side effects?
> ➤ How do you plan to come off your fast and return to eating regular food?

Why You Are Fasting?

Why you are conducting a green smoothie fast is as important as the fast itself. Having clarity around why you are doing this will support you in going the distance, whether one day or 60 days or 35 days, as was my case. My clarity was using food as medicine to eradicate the cause of a systemic skin condition that I had. I knew how long I was committed for, and I made sure my schedule would accommodate me. I already had a blender and was happy *starting where I was at* with organic and conventional produce that I purchased. And I decided that I was going to take vacation time, allowing me time to become accustomed to this process. This kept me focused, motivated and inspired—all of which I needed to help me stay the course.

Once you've established why you want to conduct a green smoothie fast and have clarity around that, the next step is deciding how long you want to fast for. In answering this question, there are a few factors that must be taken into consideration.

Any commitments that will interrupt your plan. I cleared my social schedule of anything to do with eating out; this included business and social dinners and luncheons. During my 35-day fast I attended one dinner party at the home of very close friends, and—you got it—I took my smoothie with me. "Have Mason jar, will travel!"

You may not have the luxury of not having to work through your green smoothie fast. Short-term and long-term fasts each have their own set of challenges for the working person. But the challenges are not insurmountable.

If you are undertaking a three-day or more green smoothie fast, starting on a Friday has invaluable benefits. As your body goes through the detoxification and cleansing process, you will be in the comfort of your own home. Better yet, if you are committed to a four-day or more green smoothie fast, start on a three-day weekend. This allows you to become comfortable with the process. You will be able to ascertain how much of your green smoothie you need to feel satisfied, whether you like it thick or thin, sweeter or more savory, etc.

Did you know that you don't have to make your smoothies the day you consume them? You can prepare them up to four days in advance. This is helpful if you have a busy schedule. My personal preference was to make my smoothies two days in advance. I tried four days, and for me the smoothies didn't have the same vitality as on day one or two. But it's important to know where and how you will store them.

Having all the right equipment is vital to your success. While a high-speed blender is definitely preferable, as with organic and non-organic foods, *start where you are at!* Use the blender that you have or that is within your budget. If you don't have a Vitamix or a Ninja, Cuisinart etc., this simply means that instead of putting larger pieces of fruit and vegetables into the jug, you will need to do just a little more prep work. You will need to chop your fruits and veggies up into smaller pieces. Having on hand six to nine 32-ounce (one-quart) Mason jars with lids, gives you the ideal container to drink from, and to carry and store your green smoothie in. A small cooler with an ice pack is ideal for transporting your green smoothies. This is what I use and it works well.

Start where you are at! Whether you create your green smoothie with organic or conventionally grown produce is a matter of choice. What is important is that you start the process and go the distance. I repeat, *start where you are at.*

Adding Sweeteners

Adding natural sweeteners when creating your green smoothie is optional. There are many natural sweeteners to choose from including, but not limited to, coconut sugar, maple syrup, raw honey, brown rice, and my personal choices, agave and Medjool dates. Check out your local health-food store. You may experience the desire to add a sweetener to your green smoothie when you first start drinking them. As time goes by your palate will change, and the natural sweetness of the fruits and vegetable will be enough. In fact, you may find added sweeteners too much. But until you arrive at that point, add naturally occurring sweeteners to your smoothies.

Do Not Use Artificial Sweeteners. They Are Toxic

A crucial part of your preparatory work to ensure the success of your green smoothie fast, and/or the inclusion of green smoothies into your dietary lifestyle, is letting your loved ones, friends, and work colleagues know that you are making some changes. How much you choose to explain is up to you. But it's imperative that you let everyone know that for the next XYZ days you will be conducting a green smoothie fast and therefore will not be eating regular food.

Make sure you ask everyone to support you by not bringing home your favorite ice cream, doughnuts, fried chicken, barbecue, pie, cake, etc. Don't assume that they are psychic and will know not to do this. You must communicate what your needs are so that everyone understands and is familiar with the process you are about to go through. Remember, they will be experiencing your fast right along with you. Failure to carry out these steps opens you up for self-sabotage.

To communicate effectively, it's important that you have clarity surrounding every aspect of your green smoothie fast. Duration, when you will start, the type of produce you will use, the blender you will use, how you will store your smoothies, what side effects you may encounter. Equally important is how you will reenter the world of solid foods. Having clarity around these things will make your communication to others clear, enable you to answer questions, if necessary, and allay the fears of your loved ones.

Being an introvert, I didn't tell anyone outside of my husband and sister that I was conducting a long term green smoothie fast. I elected to keep a low profile by canceling and declining all social invites. A couple of my girl friends were a more than a little hurt because I kept refusing to meet with them. Eventually, I realized if I was to keep some of those relationships intact, I needed to explain what I was doing. By then I could answer all the questions that they had, and field all the objections that I felt would have derailed me.

If you are an introvert or you prefer not to discuss your personal life with others, I suggest that you have a prepared answer for the questions and the concerns that people will have. This is a proactive supportive strategy that can go a long way to preventing you from becoming derailed from your course.

Drink Water

Drinking water is important to support your body in its elimination process. Upon awakening, the first thing you drink is 32 ounces of room-temperature pure spring water, with or without lemon. Be sure to drink several glasses of pure room temperature water throughout the day as you fast. This will help the body to detoxify without headaches and nausea.

Checking In With Your Medical Professional

When undertaking a green smoothie fast it's vitally important that you work with your health professional if you are unsure, and if you are under the care of a physician. Not to do so can put you at risk.

Q: How long can I fast for?

A: As long as you are healthy enough, you can fast for as long as you want.

Q: Can I live just on green smoothies?

A: I don't advise being on a liquid diet indefinitely without medical supervision.

Q: Do I need to prepare for my fast?

A: Yes. Preparation is important. It will support you in creating a road map for success.

Q: Can I sweeten my green smoothie?

A: Yes. You can add naturally occurring sweeteners like honey, agave, dates, maple syrup, etc.

CHAPTER 12

DETOXIFICATION, CLEANSING, & HEALING

Whether you elect to conduct a one-day or 60-day green smoothie fast, your body will go through a detoxification, cleansing and healing process. The longer your green smoothie fast is, the greater the detoxification, cleansing and healing you will experience. As you read earlier, fasting promotes your intrinsic healing response.

When your body is in cleansing and detox mode, it naturally and automatically brings to the surface impurities to be eliminated. These impurities have been wreaking havoc with your organ efficiency, healthy cell reproduction, mental clarity, vitality, and strength. Green smoothie fasting has the power to cleanse and detoxify every cell that makes up your body. And as a result, energy used to hold marauding bacteria, viruses, and microbes at bay can now be utilized for the healing and healthy regeneration of your cells.

What To Expect When Cleansing & Detoxifying

Within the first four plus days, you will experience intense detoxification. Some people experience intense purging during days three to four, and others for a little longer. During my 35-day green smoothie fast, my detoxification lasted ten days, tapering off as time went by. I can laugh now, but during the first ten days, I needed to replenish my green leafy vegetables. To do this I went to Sam's Club or

Costco to buy some organic spinach. Part of my elimination syndrome was extreme muscular fatigue. I felt like I was coming down with a bad viral flu.

At the front of the store are located power chairs for customers with mobility challenges. Believe me when I say, as I passed the chairs all lined up like soldiers, all with my name written on them, I paused, looking longingly and lovingly at each one. I took a deep breath, told myself, *No you don't, Wendy!*, and grabbed a rickety shopping cart. It was only pride that kept me out of the chair and slumped over the handle of the shopping cart as I shuffled through the store.

As your body cleanses and detoxifies it triggers your natural survival mechanism, eliminating anything that it considers to be harmful. This is what I call, "the elimination syndrome." I call it a syndrome, because, while you may experience many of the common things associated with a body cleanse and detox, your experience is going to be unique to you. This makes it a syndrome. You will have your own interpretation on how your cleansing and detoxification leaves you feeling. You may experience some or none of the reported effects or you may experience something totally new. People have reported experiencing physiological, psychological, and spiritual elimination.

Here are some of the more common effects people have experienced:-

- Diarrhea
- Constipation
- Nausea
- Headache
- Chills
- Fatigue
- Flu-like symptoms
- Doziness
- Irritability
- Mood swings
- Disinterest
- Unhappiness
- Crying jags
- Lethargy

- Loss of appetite
- Hot sweats
- Cold sweats
- Anger
- Muscle fatigue
- Joint pain and swelling
- Unusual cravings
- Desire to chew
- Craving for water
- Need to go to bed
- Cold sores
- Pimples
- Bad breath
- Intense body odor

While the above list my look very unappealing and even daunting, each reaction listed above tells you that your body is doing what it does best. Your body is designed to renew and rejuvenate itself, and to maintain optimum health.

My first ten days were…rough. From day 1, I felt irritable. Day 2, I felt disconnected from self and all things and had a headache. Day 3, all I needed was a chin wart complete with hair, a pointed hat, a cackle, and a broom to fly away on. Day 4, was a dense fog. Days 5, and 6, I spent in bed, suffering freezing chills. Day 6, muscle fatigue and joint pain. Days 7-10, some relief—a lessening of all the above experiences. Days 15-20, the desire to chew was almost overwhelming. I took care of that problem by crunching ice. Your dentist may have a fit about this!

The degree of detoxing that you may experience will be in line with how toxic your body is. Because of what was going on with me physically, psychologically and emotionally, my body was very, very toxic.

Other Things To Expect

Taste and chewing go hand in hand and a little forward planning can support you in achieving your desired green smoothie fasting goals. During your fasting process, you may experience intense cravings and the overwhelming desire for certain tastes and spices. I say tastes because you maybe craving the tanginess of barbecue sauce—not the sauce itself, but how it tastes. The tang! This can be assuaged by having a smoothie made with tamarind pulp and fresh, sweet tomatoes. Doesn't sound so good? But it tastes delicious.

During my 35-day green smoothie fast, I craved the taste of sushi, so I added a sheet of nori seaweed to my smoothie. One day I plain and simply wanted curry. Indian, Thai, West Indian it didn't matter; I just wanted curry. As one of the main ingredients in curry that gives it its distinctive flavor is cumin, I added a pinch to my smoothie along with a hint of fresh ginger, and that took care of the longing. On another occasion, I thought I would go mad if I didn't have salt, I was craving it so badly. So I added a little mineral rich Celtic salt to my smoothie and upped the amount of celery in that blend and that did the trick. It took away that craving.

One of the major desires that many people experience on a long-term fast is the desire to chew. Chewing is something that we do so automatically that it has become second nature. To get over this hurdle I chose to chew on ice and that took care of the problem.

You can be as creative as you want with your ice. You can freeze some lemon juice, or even a couple of tablespoons of your smoothie, or just the fruit or vegetables that you are using in your smoothies. Just crunch on your ice cubes instead of a handful of chips when the urge hits you. If you don't like ice, you can make your smoothie chunky, so that you have solid pieces of vegetables to chew on. This can and will take care of that craving. The name of the game is to be proactive so you don't wind up self-sabotaging.

Supporting Self Through The Green Smoothie Fasting Process

It's important to support yourself while your body is detoxifying and cleansing. This can be achieved in a number of ways. Energy work from a reflexologist or acupuncturist can be particularly helpful in speeding up and assisting in the elimination process. Each therapy opens up zones and/or meridians that allow your innate healing energy to flow smoothly. Each therapy boosts and supports the immune system and helps to lessen the impact of the natural side effects associated with green smoothie fasting.

Massage, reiki, and healing touch can help you to relax into the process and support your body as it cleanses and eliminates. It is a good idea to take an enema or schedule an appointment for a colonic at the beginning of your fast. This can help alleviate the natural side effects like constipation, diarrhea, headaches, nausea, lethargy, etc., that are associated with detoxification and cleansing. And it supports the natural healing response.

An aromatherapy and Epsom salt bath or foot soak can also help to alleviate some of the icky feeling associated with green smoothie fasting. Reconnecting with nature by walking or sitting in outdoor spaces is also helpful, as is taking the time to meditate and contemplate your life. In general, be loving to yourself. Be gentle with yourself. Take this time to get to know yourself. And above all be in gratitude for the entire process.

Detoxifying is a good thing. It must not be misconstrued as something bad, even though from personal experience it can be a little rough and leave you feeling like crap. It is getting rid of all the junk that has accumulated in your body, so that your natural healing response can work unfettered to rejuvenate your cells and maintain optimal health.

What made me keep on going even when I felt like crap? The answer to this is a little challenging for me to put into words, so I'm going to use an analogy. I hope it works. Even though there were days when I really could have used a motorized chair to take me where I wanted to go, I was intensely aware of an underlying feeling, like a vibrating, shiny, silver thread of energy that was running through the core of me. And I wanted to get to it. I wanted to get to that silver, shining core. And I knew what I had to go through to get to it. I had to go through all the junk and toxicity to get to my inner healthy core.

Perhaps a better way to describe this feeling is this: It's a beautiful sunny day. It's absolutely gorgeous and unseasonably warm. It's fall, and the leaves on the trees are turning all shades of orange and golden brown. The meteorologist on the local TV station said that the current high temperatures are abnormal. That doesn't stop the day from being glorious, or you from partaking of the gift it has given you this day. Clear blue skies with sun rays that are bright and warm, yet within the warm, gentle breeze you can feel the cool nip of winter and what's to come. It's that kind of feeling. You have to go through fall to get to winter. You have to go through a season and all that it brings to get to your favorite time of year. I knew I had to go through it to get to it!

Detoxification is not pleasant. But it really is worth it in the end. The experience, which is for a short period of time, is outweighed by the new lease on life you will have.

Q. Will I have a detox experience?
A. Yes. Although some people's experience is very mild.
Q. Is there anything I can do to stop the detoxification process?
A. No. You can support yourself through the process, but you will not be able to stop it. Supporting yourself with energy work can take the edge off the intensity of the side effects.
Q. Do I have to have an enema or colonic?
A. No, although this can help lessen some of the natural beneficial side affects (detoxing) associated with green smoothie fasting.
Q. What should I do if I feel very ill?
A. See your physician or health care provider.
Q. When does the elimination syndrome kick in?
A. Anywhere from day one to day three. Remember, your experience will be unique to you.
Q. How long will the detox and cleansing last?
A. Remembering that you are having a unique experience, this could be from one day to ten or eleven. In my case, it was a ten-day process. For many of my clients it lasted just two or three days.

CHAPTER 13
COMING OFF YOUR GREEN SMOOTHIE FAST

This is the primary reason I have written this book. Coming off of your green smoothie fast is as important as fasting itself. After drinking 64 – 96 fluid ounces of fruits, nuts and vegetables per day, you can make yourself very, very ill if breaking your fast is done incorrectly. I found this out firsthand.

When I was researching green smoothie fasting, I was surprised and a little bit puzzled that I couldn't find very much information on what you do to end your fast.

There is a rule of thumb that suggests for every ten days of fasting you need five days to reacquaint yourself with eating solid food. For three days, you need one and a half days; two days, one day and for a one-day fast, you require one-half day for integration back to eating solid food. Basically, you require half of your chosen fasting time to get back to eating your regular diet.

My green smoothie fast lasted 35 days. What this meant was that for 35 days the only thing that I ate or drank, as the case may be, was my life-giving green smoothies. Using the rule of thumb, I required 17½ days to reacquaint and integrate myself with eating and digesting solid raw and cooked food without any disastrous disruptions. And believe me, after my experience, which you will read about, I took the time limit set seriously. I chose not to rush this process. And that is my suggestion to you: Don't rush!

So, based on the limited research available coupled with my knowledge as a holistic practitioner, I figured that after 30 days, I would start out by eating a small bowl of Buddha's soup. When I say "small"—2 tablespoons, which is 60 milliliters or one fluid ounce. Buddha's soup is a simple broth made from soybean paste and slightly wilted vegetables. As I was cooking the soup, which took less than ten minutes, I was salivating. I couldn't wait to eat something hot and cooked. It's amazing the tricks we play on ourselves with the self-talk that we do. I had been telling myself that I needed to eat something cooked, because I hadn't eaten anything cooked in so long that it was a little abnormal.

As I ate the first spoonful, there were many things that I experienced, but the most profound thought I had was that the food tasted a little dead. When compared to my green smoothies, it was lifeless. There was no vitality, no vibrant energy. I said to myself, *Wenz, if you are what you eat…then this lifeless food is going to be a problem.* Once you have eaten food consisting of only raw fruit, vegetables and nuts you will totally understand what I mean when I say that the food tasted DEAD.

I was deeply disappointed. Somewhere inside me, I acknowledge that I was a little panicked, because a paradigm shift had taken place, and I didn't know what was beyond that. It was the fear of the unknown that had me in its tight grip. As I continued to eat, I realized that something wasn't right. In fact, something was terribly wrong. I finished one small bowl of soup, and against my better judgment, I talked myself into having another small bowl because, "it would taste better." It didn't! And at that point, my body rebelled. I broke out into a cold sweat and began to shake uncontrollably and then experienced horrendous stomach and intestinal cramps.

I felt as if I was experiencing food poisoning. And in a way, as I think about it now, I guess I was. In short I felt like crap! Much worse than I did when I was detoxifying. I didn't know what to do. Whether to take the drastic, unhealthy step of making myself throw up or ride it out. I just didn't know. Inducing vomiting is never, ever the way to go, so I chose to ride the storm by falling back on my spiritual training. I began focusing on my breathing, calming myself and going into a meditative state. The whole experience left me very, very, very frightened and shaken.

I didn't expect what happened to happen. I had expected the transition, starting out by eating broth, to go smoothly, and from there, to have an easy transition into eating my normal food. Because of what had happened, I immediately went back on my green smoothie fast. And for the next five days, I began to plan in detail how I was going to break my fast.

Three days after my aborted attempt I decided to break my fast by eating raw fruits, vegetables, and nuts. Instead of blending my fruits, nuts, and veggies, they would be in a bowl or on a plate. It was during this time that I realized meat was also permanently off the menu for me. Seafood and fish have worked out to be okay in small quantities, but moo the cow is...gone along with all other farm animals.

I also made the decision that for the next 17½ days, whatever I ate would be organic. This choice was prompted by the fact that I didn't want my body to have to deal with processing harsh herbicides and fertilizers that are used on most conventionally grown produce.

Remember guys, this is my experience. Each one of us is unique and therefore will experience things differently. Don't forget, start where you are at!

My first solid meal was one-third of a ripe banana, sliced, one sliced strawberry, and two walnut halves. It was delicious, and I didn't have an adverse reaction; however, I was still very timid about eating. I continued to have 64 ounces of green smoothie daily.

For five days, I ate the same thing. On the sixth day, I increased the fruit to half a banana, two strawberries, and a few raw cashew nuts. On the seventh day, I had four julienned carrots, with a little cucumber and celery. I ate only those fruits, vegetables, and nuts that I had been blending for my smoothies. This felt right and above all, safe, for me, and my body was tolerating this.

Approximately ten days into my integration back into eating solid food, I made the choice to venture a little further outside the box. I decided to make a seaweed roll using my trusted julienned veggies with a little avocado. From there, I graduated to fresh spring rolls using rice paper with lettuce, cilantro, mint, spring onions, avocado, and my trusted julienned veggies. By day 17, I was eating cooked quinoa; everything else was still raw.

From there, I went on to eating steamed, curried, and stir-fried vegetables. My integration process took nearly 30 days, because that's what I needed. Be guided by what your body is telling you. Don't force the process.

Keys For Coming Off Your Fast:

- ✓ Using the rule of thumb, calculate the length of your integration process
- ✓ Drink at least one 32-ounce green smoothie daily
- ✓ Decide if you want to eat two, three, or four tiny meals consisting of fruit and/or vegetables.
- ✓ Begin eating very, very small amounts of fruit, and, if you included nut milks into your smoothie, use those nuts. Example: less than a third of a banana, a sliver of melon, a quarter of a mango, and two nuts. Work your way over the course of your calculated integration time into consuming the whole fruit.
- ✓ Switch to eating a very small serving of vegetables i.e. a quarter of a carrot, a little celery or cucumber.
- ✓ Drink plenty of water.
- ✓ Use mineral rich Celtic sea salt or sea salt.
- ✓ Work your way over the course of your calculated integration time into eating lightly cooked vegetables.
- ✓ Lightly steam vegetable so they are *al dente*. They can be served with a sprinkling of fresh herbs.
- ✓ Add steamed rice or quinoa.
- ✓ Stir-fry in coconut oil (again so that vegetables are *al dente*), use wheat- and sugar-free soy sauce, onion, garlic, etc.
- ✓ Include when breaking your fast lots of fresh salads with citrus vinaigrette.
- ✓ Once you have completed your calculated integration process, you can add meat, fish, and dairy back into your diet.
- ✓ Follow the Dietary Principle.

If you find that eating a certain food causes you nausea, my suggestion would be to eliminate it from your diet—even if it was your favorite thing to eat before you went on your green smoothie fast. If you find yourself craving green smoothies or totally satisfied with more green smoothies than solid food, follow your wishes.

If your palate has changed and you find yourself embracing more of a live raw food diet, then go with that. This is where I am at. My preference is to eat raw fruits, nuts, and vegetables, although, traveling outside my home environment has brought me the gift of, albeit forced, flexibility.

Q. Can I start eating regular food when I've completed my green smoothie fast?
A. No! To prevent yourself from becoming violently ill and feeling like CRAP, you must integrate back to eating regular food slowly. Your body and digestive system need time to adjust.
Q. Should I eat lots of small meals or one large meal?
A. Your meals should graduate from tiny, to small, to your regular-size portions. Eating too much in one sitting can cause you to feel really unwell.
Q. If I'm more comfortable drinking just green smoothies can I do that?
A. I would caution against living on a liquid diet for the rest of your life unless supervised by a physician. You can include green smoothies as part of your diet.

CHAPTER 14
TRAVELING & GREEN SMOOTHIES

Traveling as a serious green smoothie drinker and a predominately raw-foodist, even with planning, can be a challenge. If you are traveling and have elected to be a guest in someone's home, it is in your best interest to make sure that you have the run of the kitchen. I have decided that if I am invited to stay in someone's home as a guest, I'm going to give my hosts a gift of a high-speed blender. That way I have the major piece of equipment that I need in order to eat the way in which I want. And my hosts have a wonderful thank-you gift. At the end of the day, a high-speed blender—Vitamix, Blendtec, Ninja— is approximately the cost of a two- or three-night stay at a hotel.

Many people understand vegetarianism and the desire not to eat meat or fish. But you'll find that many have a hard time not understanding the nuances associated with the desire not to eat processed or prepackaged foods…even those that are touted to be "healthy." The minute you express your dietary lifestyle, people get really, really, really panicked. The question you'll be asked is, "So what do you eat?"

My response is, "I eat fruits, vegetables, nuts, and grains. Sugar free, wheat free and gluten free products. I have an allergy to wheat and sugar." LOL! Then they'd ask, "Oh...so, what do you eat?"

I found out that being a pescetarian actually solved many challenges while I was away. Let's just say everyone was happy (in their comfort zone) to fry, pan sear, steam, or stew fish and serve it with steamed vegetables.

Plan your travel carefully; it will cut down on stress associated with eating in the way that you want. Find out beforehand if you will have access to organic produce or a local farmers markets etc. If not, have a plan B. As I mentioned earlier, your hostess gift can be the equipment you need to survive, so that will not be a problem. You can also support yourself by traveling with dehydrated foods, nuts, and homemade granola.

Q: What do I do if I'm traveling?
A: Forward planning is key to your success. Conduct a little research into what produce is available along with amenities to create your Green Is 4 Life smoothie.

In addition to gifting your hosts with a high-speed blender, you can also purchase a bullet, which is designed to make a small (12 – 16-ounce) smoothie and is light enough to travel with. However, because of the blades you will have check your bag.

CHAPTER 15
IN A NUTSHELL, WHAT DO I DO TO FAST?

The points below highlight the things you need to do when going on a green smoothie fast.

➤ Make a choice to commit to fasting.
➤ Decide on the length of time you want to fast for and commit to it. (See chapter 11.)
➤ Make sure you are healthy enough to conduct a fast. Check with your health-care professional before undertaking a fast.
➤ Make sure you have the equipment needed to create your smoothies. (See chapter 25.)
➤ If possible, start your fast on the Friday before a two- or three-day weekend.
➤ Let people know that you aren't eating regular food. Allay their fears by letting them know that veggies will give you all the nutrients you need to maintain excellent health.
➤ If cooking for your family, plan your meals in advance.
➤ Drink a smoothie while cooking.
➤ Drink a smoothie when sitting down to eat with friends and family.
➤ If you are working during your fast, prepare your green smoothies up to four days in advance. (Personal preference here is two days in advance.)
➤ Take 32 ounces of water with you when you retire for the night, and drink it first thing in the morning.
➤ Try not to drink your smoothie straight out of the refrigerator; give it ten or fifteen minutes at room temperature.
➤ Keep the smoothie in your mouth for about five seconds before swallowing.

➤ Be prepared for the detoxification symptoms you may experience. (See chapter 12.)

➤ Have a cooler in which to transport your smoothies and/or your prepared greens, fruits and vegetables. (See chapter 14.)

➤ Rotate greens, fruits, and vegetables. (See chapter 18.)

➤ Use nut, seed and grain milks and coconut water in your smoothies.

➤ Sweeten, if necessary, with natural sweeteners. (See chapter 20.)

➤ Support your body, mind, and spirit through the process. (See chapter 12.)

➤ Come off your fast slowly, integrating back into eating solid by eating tiny bowls of fruit. (See chapter 13.)

➤ Have a plan for reintegration to eating normal food. (See chapter 13.)

➤ Be patient with yourself and others.

➤ *Start where you are at!*

Planning! Planning! Planning! Planning is the most vital part of conducting a fast and including daily green smoothies into your dietary lifestyle.

CHAPTER 16
INTEGRATING GREEN SMOOTHIES INTO YOUR CURRENT DIETARY LIFESTYLE

So you are not going to do a green smoothie fast, but you want them as a part of your life? Integrating life-giving green smoothies into your current dietary lifestyle is relatively simple. Once again, *start where you are at!* The inclusion of green smoothies into your life can give you many of the benefits of fasting, but at a much slower pace. However, many people have reported that in just three weeks they are experiencing a boost of energy, more restful sleep and a reduction in cravings. Some people have even experienced weight loss. And this is by drinking anything from 16 to 32 fluid ounces daily.

Much like fasting, the inclusion of green smoothies into your diet starts by you making a conscious choice and commitment to do so.

How Do I Include Green Smoothie Into My Lifestyle?

Adding 16 - 32 ounces of green smoothie into your current dietary life style is all about inclusion and integration. The inclusion of raw fruits, vegetables and green leafy vegetables with nuts, seeds, grains and herbs in the form of a nutritious drink, is just that, inclusion. It has nothing to do with removing or excluding any foods that you are currently eating. On the contrary, it's about expanding and adding to your current food horizon.

When I first witnessed the demonstration for Vitamix and Blendtec, I was enthralled…and on some level, I continue to be. These demonstrators where all instrumental in helping me to coin the phrase, "Start where you are at." In their demonstrations, complete with earpiece and microphone, the flamboyant and smooth- talking demonstrators used little pieces of leftover vegetables, whose refrigerator life- expectancy was zero. You know, like the end of a cucumber, a bit of carrot, a quarter of an apple, a couple of strawberries, some frozen organic mixed vegetables (available at Costco), fruit juice, half a banana, and a peach, minus the stone, that needed to be used up and a few cups of ice. They blended these at a high speed to make a delicious, nutritious smoothie.

What the demonstrators told me equated to, "Start where you are at!" Start with what you have on hand. If you currently have any vegetables, frozen or otherwise, in your refrigerator, use them. If you have some fruit—fresh and/or frozen— include it. Let's say in your refrigerator you currently have a bit of zucchini, some carrots, a cucumber, and a bit of lettuce or spinach or even cabbage. Maybe you also have corn, green peas or beans or oats, and fruit juice. Put them in your blender with ice and/or water, a little honey or agave to taste, and a smattering of herbs or spices. Hit the blend switch, and you have just created a nutritious green smoothie. You've also saved money by using up fruits and veggies that would have gone to waste.

If drunk on a regular basis, your green smoothie drink will change your life. It's really as simple as that.

Recently while on vacation, I used the simple principle below to support my green smoothie lifestyle. I couldn't always get what I wanted, so I purchased a bag of frozen mixed vegetables. Would this have been my first choice? No! It wouldn't. However, based on my circumstances it was a brilliant option. You see, "I started where I was at."

Just as an FYI: When selecting your produce, fruits, vegetables, nuts, seeds and grains you are always looking for freshness and organically grown. With that in mind my suggested order of preference to create your Green Is 4 Life smoothie is as follows:

Organic grown fresh (pick your own).
Organic co-operative baskets.

Conventionally grown farm-fresh (pick your own).
Conventionally grown.
Organic flash-frozen.
Conventionally flash-frozen.
Glass jar, organic.
Glass jar, conventionally grown.

Then and only then after exhausting all the other options, would you use tinned veggies and fruits. And as much as possible make sure they are organic, too.

Suggested Order of Preference for Purchasing Produce

There is a theory that simply states, "Consuming food that is locally grown and harvested helps you to support and maintain a healthy immune system." My suggested purchasing order is as follows:

Locally grown organic.
From surrounding areas/regional organic.
From the same country organic.
Imported. (Some produce like coconuts, mangos and other exotic fruits and vegetables will always be imported, as they are not native to the country that you live in. This is true of other fruits and vegetables.)

Including Green Smoothies Into Your Dietary Lifestyle

Here are some of the ways that you can include and integrate green smoothies into your current dietary lifestyle. Your Green Is 4 Life smoothies can be eaten:-

➢ As a meal
➢ Or in conjunction with your meal.
➢ As a cold soup
➢ As a liquid salad
➢ With dessert

- ➢ In place of your dessert
- ➢ To replace energy boost drinks that are designed to keep you going
- ➢ As a snack
- ➢ When eating on the run
- ➢ As a time saver when you don't have time to prepare a meal, but need something substantial to eat
- ➢ If you just don't feel like cooking
- ➢ As a balanced meal replacement for the elderly
- ➢ To build strength
- ➢ To support rebuilding of strength after an illness
- ➢ When you don't have the desire to cook for one person

As you see, there are numerous ways in which to include life-giving green smoothies into your current lifestyle.

As you know yourself best, I have a question I want to ask: What does it look like for you to include a daily green smoothie in your dietary lifestyle?

If it looks like a lot of work...then you are not starting where you are at. While I am not advocating this, as this book is called *Green Is 4 Life,* some of my clients have had to work their way into adding the "green" bit of the green smoothie into their blend. And this is fine also. They have essentially elected to drink a daily smoothie that is mostly fruit, with cucumber and/or lettuce. *Start where you are at.* The most important thing is that you start and continue. You can build from that point...even if you want to make your smoothie with yoghurt.

CHAPTER 17
YOGHURT-BASED SMOOTHIES

By now, I know that you know my mantras, "Start where you are at!" And "Do your own due diligence." A large percentage of my clientele base uses yoghurt as the base for their smoothies. The yoghurt takes the place of water and/or nut, grain, or seed milks.

While it's fair to say that I do have some strong arguments against drinking milk and eating yoghurt, I recognize that they are my thoughts and feelings, and it's totally unfair to impress them upon you. What I would say is, please *do your own due diligence*. Research the pros and cons of drinking milk-based products.

That being said, I have a couple of suggestions I would like to offer. In fact, I have four things to which I would like you to give every consideration.

Purchase yoghurt that has been made from cows that are organically fed and humanely treated. Eat yoghurt made from milk that has been put through a low-heat pasteurization process. Straus is the brand that I suggest. This is found at most large health-food stores. You can also ask your local grocery store to carry it, and that includes asking Wal-Mart and Target...you never know, they just may accommodate you.

Use plain yoghurt kefir instead of the normal yoghurt that you buy. Some major grocery stores and international food markets carry this product. If not your local larger health-food store will have it.

Make your own yoghurt using low-heat pasteurized organic milk with milk kefir grains or yoghurt starter. The milk kefir is really the way to go. Yes, it's a process, but it's so worth it. Check out milk kefir and the whole yoghurt making process on YouTube. In the search box, type "milk kefir" and see all the wonderful information that comes up.

Try using nut, seed, or grain milks: almond, hazelnut, Brazil nut, and my favorite, cashew nut milk. Or milk from grains: oats, hemp, rice, or soy blended with banana, papaya, or avocado to create a delicious substitute for your yoghurt.

You will experience several of the benefits associated with the inclusion of a daily green smoothie into your current dietary practices, especially when using yoghurt kefir. Kefir is a live culture that balances your naturally occurring intestinal flora, supporting your internal ecology and promoting better digestion.

I don't suggest fasting with yoghurt. I feel that your digestive track will have to work too hard during the assimilation and absorption process. Remember with green smoothie fasting, you will be consuming between 64 and 96 fluid ounces of smoothie per day. If you include yoghurt, more energy will be used in the digestion of the animal-based protein, leaving less to trigger the healing response.

Q: Can I use yoghurt for my green smoothie fasting?
A: NO! To conduct a green smoothie fast, you will need to make the transition to nut milks and coconut or soy yoghurt.
Q: Can I use yoghurt to incorporate green smoothies into my daily eating practices?
A: Yes. But remember you will be drinking between 16 and 32 ounces daily and the digestive tract has to work hard to process animal-based foods.

CHAPTER 18
ROTATING YOUR GREENS

It's also important to rotate the fruit, vegetables, and green leafy vegetables that you use to create your nutritious green smoothies.

I love, love, love spinach. I could eat it daily. And as a result of that love affair, in my early fasting days I would put spinach in nearly all of my Green Is 4 Life smoothies. And during my 35-day green smoothie fast, spinach was initially my green leaf of choice. After drinking spinach for nearly ten days in a row, my body started to rebel. When I put the Mason jar to my mouth to take a healthy swallow of my smoothie, my mouth, throat, and stomach said, "Hell no! See what we'll do if you try to take a swallow of that stuff!" I was drinking over 96 fluid ounces a day, and my green leafy vegetable of choice was spinach. I could pack in a whopping 12 to 16 ounces—or more!—of spinach.

It dawned on me that somewhere in my research, I had come across a statement that suggested that when conducting a green smoothie fast or adding green smoothies to your diet, you need to ensure that you rotate your fruits, veggies, and green leafy vegetables.

It has been suggested the oxalic acid present in plants, if over-eaten, can trigger a kind of temporary allergenic response, much like I experienced with the spinach. Or it's like the way over-stuffing yourself on a favorite food can sometime lead to the very *thought* of that food's making you feel physically ill.

I learned three major things from the experience of not following through with fruit and veggie rotation.

Firstly, whoever has written that piece of information was totally correct. You MUST rotate your veggies, in particular your green leafy vegetables.

The second intriguing snippet of understanding that I came away with is that everything in nature has a way of ensuring the survival of the species. Plants have their own chemical defense mechanism. It's called oxalic acid. Each plant has its own level of oxalic acid. When combined with other unique characteristics it creates a dynamic that keeps insects at bay and prevents grazing animals from eating a plant into extinction.

The same survival mechanism applies when we overeat a plant. What we experience first is an aversion to the food we are consuming, like what happened to me when I was eating so much spinach in my green smoothies. Should we continue eating, we experience gas, bloating, and nausea, and then a mild allergic response. From there, we may go on to full-blown disorders and diseases. Many people are already at the stage where the food that they are consuming on a daily basis is creating gas and bloating or an allergic response. The next stage is the creation of chronic dis-ease.

In our green smoothies, we are able to use green leafy vegetables on a daily bases, because each plants defense mechanism is made up of more than oxalic acid. Components that are unique to each plant are also involved in the defense process. This is why we are able to use different green leafy vegetables on a daily bases and suffer no allergic reaction.

My third bit of wisdom was to pay attention to boredom. Boredom is the first sign from your body that you need to do something different because what you are doing isn't working out for you. The emotional feeling of boredom gives you the heads-up that you are getting ready to self-sabotage. Different greens bring something new and exciting to the table in the way of flavor, texture, and nutritional value.

From nature, we can learn so much. Grazing cattle and foraging animals continuously move from place to place. They know that they can't overeat a particular plant, because the survival mechanism in that plant won't let them. In moving around, they look for a variety of plants, because each has something essential to offer in the way of nutrients and micronutrients.

And so it is with you. You are looking for the highest infusion of nutrients, micronutrients and trace minerals with every green smoothie consumed. In order to achieve that state, you must rotate your green leafy vegetables.

On a personal note, because of the crucial rotation factor in creating the perfect green smoothie, it's very rare that I mix more than two types of greens together in my creation. This allows me to have a wider variety to choose from and prevents me from maxing out on choices. It also keeps me within the rotation factor. When I do mix my greens, I usually choose to add dandelions, watercress, or mustard greens to the mix. For me, the above mentioned have a very strong flavor by themselves, so I have chosen to use them in a mix.

Q: Do I have to rotate my green leafy vegetables?
A: Yes. Otherwise, you can quickly build an intolerance to them.
Q: Do I have to rotate my fruits, vegetables, and nut milks?
A: Yes. While you can have a longer run with consuming the same fruits, vegetables, and nuts, failure to rotate will eventually cause you to build up an intolerance.
Q: How will I know if I am building up an intolerance?
A: Your green smoothie will be very, very, very unappealing!
Q: Are there any other signs I should look for?
A: Yes: gas and bloating, followed by a wave of nausea.
Q: How long does it take for the intolerance to go away?
A: Once you've rotated your greens, you should be fine.

CHAPTER 19
NUT, GRAIN & SEED MILKS

Nut, seed, and grain milks are a delicious and nutritious way of adding the fluid needed to create your green smoothies. All nut and grain milks are enriched with naturally occurring fiber and protein, as well as vitamins and minerals, all of which are added to your smoothie-making equation. Iron, zinc, manganese, calcium, folic acid, magnesium, vitamin B complex, vitamin E, potassium, trace minerals like copper etc., are the building blocks of health and healthy cell regeneration.

Nuts and grains also have their own uniqueness of flavor, personality, depth, tone, smell, and texture. All of this helps you to create a customized green smoothie that will be pleasing to your palate.

Nut, seed, and grain milks are relatively easy to make. The equipment is a high-speed blender, nut-milk bag or cheesecloth or extra-fine sieve, and a sterile 32-ounce Mason jar or 950-milliliter Kilner jar. Each recipe make approximately 32oz, 4 cups, or 1 liter.

Sterilizing Your Mason Jars

Sterilizing your Mason jars are an easy process and it helps to preserve your milk. If your dishwasher has that function, you can use that. If not, wash your jars in hot soapy water, rinse well. Fill a pot with water large enough to submerge jars. When water is boiling, submerge Mason jars and boil for 10 – 20 minutes. Remove with tongs and allow to drain and cool. Your jars are now ready to be used. To store sterilized jars cover with clean lids and keep in a dust free environment. To avoid burns and injury, please use caution when using hot water. **FYI**: Be sure to pit your dates; and check store bought pitted dates too, otherwise the stone will damage your blender.

Oat Milk

1 cup (8 fl. oz., 227g.) oats, soaked overnight, rinsed, and strained (old fashion oat)
4 cups (32 fl. oz., 950 ml) water
5 – 6 pitted dates (Be sure to pit your dates; and check store bought pitted dates too otherwise the stone will damage your blender) or 2 tablespoons (1 fl. oz., 30 ml) sweetener of your choice (optional, see chapter 20 for information on sweeteners)

Place all ingredients in blender, and put on the lid. Blend/blitz until smooth and creamy.

Place nut-milk bag, cheesecloth, or extra-fine sieve over a non-reactive bowl. Pour oat mixture through and gently squeeze the milk out. Once you are unable to get any more milk through, you are done!

Pour your oat milk into a clean and sterile Mason jar. Keep in your refrigerator. Your milk will last for approximately 3 – 4 days. Shake before using.

Brown Rice Milk

1 cup (8 oz., 227g.) cooked long-grain brown rice
3 – 4 cups (24 – 32 fl. oz., 700 – 950 ml) water
6 pitted dates or 2 tablespoons (1 fl. oz., 30 ml) or sweetener of your choice (optional, see chapter 20 for information on sweeteners)
Pinch salt (optional)

Place all the ingredients in blender, and put on the lid. Blend/blitz until smooth and creamy.

Place nut-milk bag, cheesecloth, or extra-fine sieve over a non-reactive bowl. Pour rice mixture through, and gently squeeze the milk out. Once you are unable to get any more milk through, you are done!

Pour your rice milk into a clean and sterile Mason jar. Keep in your refrigerator. Your milk will last for approximately 3 - 4 days. Shake before using.

Coconut Milk 1
2 cups (16 oz., 454g.) unsweetened, shredded organic coconut
6 pitted dates or 2 tbsp. (1 fl. oz., 30ml) or sweetener of your choice (optional, see chapter 20 for information on sweeteners)
4 cups (32 fl. oz., 950 ml) hot (not boiling) water
Place all ingredients in blender, and put on the lid.

Cover the lid of blender with a folded towel to prevent hot water and steam escaping and blend/blitz until smooth and creamy. The mixture will be very textured.

Let coconut mixture rest in blender for approximately 10 minutes. Place nut-milk bag, cheesecloth, or extra-fine sieve over a large non-reactive bowl. Pour nut mixture through, and when cool enough, gently squeeze the milk out. Once you are unable to get any more milk through, you are done!

Pour your coconut milk into a clean and sterile Mason jar. Keep in your refrigerator. Your milk will last for approximately 3 – 4 days. Since there are no preservatives or fillers, the "cream" of the coconut milk may separate out and rest on the top. Just shake or stir before using.

Coconut Milk 2
1 brown or white coconut with meat removed from shell
3 – 4 cups (24 –32 fl. oz., 700 – 950 ml) water
3 – 6 dates or 2 tbsp. (1 fl. oz., 30ml) or sweetener of your choice (optional, see chapter 20 for information on sweeteners)

Cut coconut into large chunks (small bite-size pieces if you are not using a high-speed blender like Vitamix, Blendtec). Or peel outer brown layer leaving white meat, and cut into chunks.

Pour the water into the blender. Add the coconut chunks, put on the lid, and blend until mixture is textured pulp.

Place nut milk bag or cheesecloth over a large non-reactive bowl. Pour nut mixture through and gently squeeze the milk out. Once you are unable to get any more milk through, you are done!

Pour your coconut milk into a clean and sterile Mason jar. Keep in your refrigerator. Your milk will last for approximately 3 – 4 days.

Since there are no preservatives or fillers, the "cream" of the coconut milk may separate out and rest on the top. Just shake or stir before using.

Almond Milk

1½ cups (12 oz., 340g.) raw organic almonds, rinsed and soaked overnight (see directions)
4 pitted dates or 2tbps. (1 fl. oz., 30 ml) or sweetener of your choice (optional, see chapter 20 for information on sweeteners)
4 cups (32 fl. oz., 950 ml) cold water
Pinch salt

Rinse almonds, then place in a non-reactive container, glass or stainless steel (I use my Mason/Kilner jar) and soak overnight or for 8 hours in 2 cups (16 fl. oz., 475ml) water.

Drain almonds and place in blender with other ingredients, and put on the lid. Blend/blitz until smooth and creamy.

Place nut-milk bag, cheesecloth, or extra-fine sieve over a non-reactive bowl. Pour nut mixture through, and gently squeeze the milk out.

NOTE: In this recipe, this step is optional. Your milk will be thicker and retain the nut fiber if you don't squeeze it.

Pour your almond milk into a clean and sterile Mason jar. Keep in your refrigerator. Your milk will last for approximately 3 – 4 days. Shake before using. Also, try the same recipe for cashews, hazelnuts, pecans, macadamia nuts, walnuts and pistachios. They are delicious. Instead of dates to sweeten, you can use honey, agave or maple syrup.

Flavored Milks

To make vanilla-flavored nut milk add 1 teaspoon of pure almond extract or ½ a vanilla bean when blending nuts and water.

To make chocolate- flavored almond milk, add 2 tablespoons of raw cocoa powder or carob powder.

Remember, always check with your health care professional before making changes to your diet.

Suggested Soak Time For Nuts & Seeds

I don't always presoak my nuts or seeds, but all nuts and seeds, with the exception of coconut, can be soaked overnight. The idea of presoaking is that the dormant nut takes in water, which triggers its sprouting response. It awakens, releases enzymes, and becomes alive. Always rinse well. Then blend with spring water to make your milk.

Do your own due diligence. Allow your experience to help you decide what works for you.

Ratios of Nuts, Seeds, & Grains to Water

Again, *do your own due diligence.* The ratio is usually 1 cup of nuts, grains, or seeds to 2 – 4 cups of water. For thicker milk, use less water; for thinner milk, use more water. You can play around to get the exact ratios that work for you.

The following are a list of nuts, seeds, and grains that you can experiment with to make delicious and nutritious milks for your green smoothie bases:

Seeds: sesame, hemp seeds, flax, pumpkin, sunflower, and pine nuts.

Nuts: cashew, hazelnut, pecans, macadamia, walnut, pistachio, almond, and coconut.

Note: Grains like rice, oats, etc. need to be strained. So does coconut. For other seed and nut milks, straining with the nut-milk bag, cheesecloth, or extra-fine sieve is optional.

Some grains, like rice and barley, need to be precooked before making milk. Others, like oats, rye, etc. need to be soaked overnight and rinsed before making milk. Have fun with the milk-making process!

CHAPTER 20
SWEETENERS

When you first start making your green smoothies you may find that you require a little sweetener to make your drink more palatable. This is fairly common and many newbies have this experience. What you'll find is that the more you drink your green smoothies with naturally-ripened fruit, the less you'll need to add sweeteners to create a palatable drink.

There are many different sweeteners available on the market. Finding out what works for you is truly a matter of personal taste. I strongly suggest, however, that you use a true natural sweetener and stay away from artificial sweeteners and table sugars.

Not All Sweeteners Are Equal

Not all sweeteners are made equal, so therefore, it's important to do your own due diligence. Educate yourself on how your chosen sweetener has been produced. For instance, honey is made by bees and collected from their hives. You can't get any more natural than that. All you have to do is squeeze the honey out of the combs, and, hey presto, you have a natural sweetener.

The question to ask yourself is "How processed is the sweetener you are currently consuming?" Has it been heat pasteurized or is it raw? Was it a low or high temperature pasteurization process? Was the sweetener mixed with any kind of corn or fructose syrup?

What does that mean for the nutritional benefits conferred on you as the consumer?

Agave nectar is another natural sweetener that I use. A naturally occurring nectar, agave is one of the main ingredients use in the production of tequila. Much like raw honey during the Roman era, agave nectar was used by the Aztecs to assist in the healing of wounds. When water is evaporated out of the nectar, it creates a sweet syrup. The thing for you to determine is whether the agave you are using has been created in a laboratory or has the nectar been harvested from an agave plant? Was the evaporation process that is needed to produce the syrup, carried out using high temperatures and or chemicals, or was it low temperature and chemical-free? Low temperature and chemical free is the product to use.

To find out how any sweetener of your choice was produced simply contact the company and ask. Educate yourself! You'll find that some of the so-called "natural" sweeteners are more processed than table sugars. Again, educate yourself so that you can make an informed decision about what you are putting into your body.

Here are some natural sweeteners for you to check out

➢ Dates (Medjool)
➢ Raw honey
➢ Agave
➢ Rapadura (raw evaporated cane sugar)
➢ Brown rice syrup
➢ Coconut palm sugar
➢ Maple syrup
➢ Molasses

"Do I start where I am at?" NO!!!! Not if you are using artificial sweeteners. In this instance, my mantra does not apply. You will need to make another selection from the list above or by going to your local health-food store and chatting with one of the knowledgeable clerks.

You may have noted that some of the more popular *natural* sweeteners are not on my list. This is because by the time the manufacturers have finished processing the raw material with an overabundance of chemicals and heat, they are no longer natural, but have become chemically laden, which equates to toxicity when consumed.

> Q: What is the best sweetener to use in a smoothie?
> A: It's a matter of personal preference.
> Q: Which sweetener would you suggest?
> A: Medjool dates. They sweeten without overpowering your green smoothie.
> Q: Can I use artificial sweeteners in my smoothie?
> A: NO! NO! NO

CHAPTER 21
PROTEIN

When people think about going on a green smoothie fast they usually ask two questions: "How will I get my protein?" and, "How will I get my calcium?"

Protein is one of the major building blocks of the human body and plays a major role in maintaining your health and well-being. Proteins are present throughout your body, providing structure and helping create important substances like the amino acids required for good health.

Protein aids in the building and repair of body tissues, the regulation of body processes, and the formation of enzymes and hormones. Protein cannot be stored by the body as can fats and carbohydrates, for later use. Protein is a necessary component of the human diet and is essential for good health.

I believe, you have been erroneously taught that the only way you can get protein and calcium is through the consumption of animal flesh and animal products, such as milk, eggs, cheese, etc. What you haven't been told, but what is known by the food industry, is that vegetables, nuts, seeds and fruits, have all the protein, minerals, trace minerals, and vitamins that you could ever need. And what's more, they are naturally packaged in a way that is easy for human consumption. They also come without all the current concerns surrounding trans fats, cholesterol, etc. that are so prevalent in processed foods.

Vegetables contain protein and vitamins in addition to trace minerals. In fact, they have all that you need to keep your body healthy and strong. Emerging research is showing that vegetables appear to contain 2.5% more protein than meat. And what's more, it's easier for the body to absorb and assimilate vegetable protein than it is meat protein.

I know based on the dietary bill of goods that we have been sold; many people feel that unless they eat meat and or dairy products they will not get the industry suggested, recommended daily amount, RDA of protein. So I have a question for you: "What are some of the largest land mammals known to man?" In answer to that question, what springs to mind are elephants and hippos.

The average male elephant is solid muscle weighing in at six to eight tons! That's a whopping 12 to 16 thousand pounds! You can get a feel for how heavy elephants are when you consider that most cars weigh approximately 2½ tons, or 5 thousand pounds. An adult elephant can consume approximately 300 pounds of fruits, grasses, barks, shrubs, roots, leaves, etc. per day. The water horse, or hippopotamus, weighs in at 5 to 8 thousand pounds (2½ to 5 tons) and can eat approximately 80 pounds of food daily. That's grasses, shrubs, roots, etc.

The point I'm making is that elephants, like hippos, rhinos, buffalos, wildebeest, cows, sheep, goats, rabbits, etc., are all herbivorous. That's right they are all vegetarians. And they are all solid muscle.

In regard to calcium and your being able to consume enough to support and maintain the health of your teeth and bones, let me allay your fears. Calcium, like protein, is present in most fruits, nuts, seeds, and vegetables. As are the B-vitamins and vitamins D, K, A, C, and E, and minerals like copper, zinc, iron, etc. Read about the nutritional value of fruits, nuts, seeds, and vegetables so you can make an educated decision on what you are choosing to eat and why.

In an earlier chapter, I stated that food is medicine. It is, for all the reasons I have cited above, in addition to the fact that nature provides you, in the form of plants, with everything you need to build and repair your body. In all plant life, you will find an abundance of "user- friendly" proteins, vitamins, minerals and trace elements, nutrients and micronutrients, along with fiber and water. Not only is a green smoothie an excellent controlled delivery system, injecting mega nutrients directly into your digestive system for optimum uptake, it's also designed to trigger your innate healing response. Furthermore, greens smoothies support you by providing you with the nutrients that you need to maintain your health physically, emotional/mentally and spiritually.

Once again, *do your own due diligence*. Be your own finder of cold, hard facts by getting your nutritional information on fruits, nuts, seeds, and vegetables. Try including green smoothies into your diet for four weeks and check in with yourself at the end of your time to see how you feel.

Q: Do I have to eat meat or cheese to get my RDA of protein?
A: No, you will get all the protein that you need from plants and fruits.
Q: Will I become deficient in protein by conducting a green smoothie fast?
A: No. By eating a good cross-section of green leafy vegetables and vegetables combined with fruits, nuts, seeds, and grains you will not become deficient in protein.
Q: Will I get all the vitamins I need from a green smoothie?
A: Yes. When your green smoothie is created using the Dietary Principle, you will get all the vitamins, minerals and trace minerals your body requires to heal and repair itself and to maintain good health.

CHAPTER 22
SENIORS & GREEN SMOOTHIES

With the passage of time all things must change, and so it is with your body. Aging is a reality, regardless of what the anti-aging commercials tell you. Some changes you experience will be the stuff that dreams are made of. The ability to say what you want without filters is one of the things that I have noticed comes with the passage of time. Another is realizing what is really important to you.

Some of the other things that accompany aging are a bit more of a challenge. Age-related diseases and disorders, the inability to chew well, the inability to digest foods you have enjoyed in the past, and chronic constipation or diarrhea just scratch the surface.

Another big problem for seniors is inability to consistently get the right nutrition that triggers the innate healing response, so that the body can repair and rejuvenate itself and maintain excellent health. The reasons for these inabilities are as varied as they are unique to each individual. You may no longer be interested in the preparation and cooking of meals. You may not be able to get out and shop the way you once did. Or maybe you are living on a fixed income, which impacts the way you eat, or you may be suffering from appetite loss. Whatever your reason it is a problem, and an industry-recognized problem at that.

So much so that in 1973, a medical nutrition product, a beverage called Ensure was launched. Ensure was formulated to provide consumers with calories, protein and essential vitamins and minerals. Ensure is intended for supplemental use with or between meals and for short-term sole-source nutrition.

Ensure products cover a wide range of categories claiming to provide a source of nutrition in connection with aging; recovery from illness, injury, or surgery; and managing physical and mental conditions that cause an inability or refusal to eat, appetite loss, or overall weight loss.

I know of many seniors who are currently using Ensure for the claim that it provides a balanced source of nutrition. My late uncle, Will Wright, was an avid Ensure drinker while he was going through chemotherapy and radiation and thereafter. I maintained then, as I still do now that Ensure DID NOT give him what he needed nutritionally to support his health in any way.

If I had known then, what I know now, things would have been done differently. And yes, this baby Rottweiler—which is what he affectionately called me—would have first ensured that Uncle Will would have been on green juices (without fiber) and then graduated up to green life-giving smoothies with fiber.

I'm not saying, and will not say, that green smoothies would have saved him. To engage in that kind of debate is futile and a total waste of energy. Green smoothies are not a panacea.

What I am saying is that the drinking of green smoothies would have triggered and supported his innate health response by injecting live, raw nutrients into his digestive system, in a way that made them readily available for the body to use. This would have positively impacted the way he felt and his energy levels, and it would have helped to trigger his natural healing response.

Green smoothies offer seniors a delicious way of getting a balanced source of nutrition packed with vitamins, minerals, trace minerals, and fiber. They provide you with a good source of protein and calories. Green smoothies are easy to prepare with a minimum of fuss. They can be used as a daily "live" vitamin. They can also be used a nutritional supplement that is eaten with or between meals. Green smoothies can be use as a meal replacement and for short-term sole-source nutrition. To ensure that you are getting all the electrolytes your body requires for healthy heart and nerve stimulus, boost your smoothie by making it with pure coconut water. Coconut is nature's natural source of electrolytes, rich in potassium, chlorides, magnesium, phosphorus and calcium, etc. (See chapter 8.)

You can prepare your smoothies for a couple days in advance, making them convenient to integrate into your life. Smoothies are easy to digest and simple to customize to suit your taste buds.

Several of my senior clients ranging from 78 to 90 years old (including my parents, who are 82 and 85) have successfully incorporated green smoothies into their current dietary life style. They make their smoothies with fresh and frozen fruits and vegetables and fresh green leafy vegetables. Many clients have elected to have their smoothies in the morning, before breakfast, as breakfast, or with breakfast. My parents, on the other hand have chosen to have their smoothies at night in place of the hot nighttime drink they used to have.

One of the things that I noticed when recently visiting my parents, who incidentally have a very healthy dietary lifestyle, is that they don't eat a lot of fat. Good fat or bad fat, they don't eat enough of it. Fat is necessary to support healthy brain function. A couple of teaspoons of coconut oil or a healthy fistful of nuts added to your smoothie will ensure that you are getting all the fat that you need for your brainpower. Are you getting enough good fats in your diet?

When incorporating green smoothies into your dietary lifestyle, start out by purchasing a few extra vegetables: spinach or your favorite greens, plus perhaps celery, carrots, and/or zucchini. Pick up some, raw nuts, and grab some fruit—bananas, apples, or whatever you see and like. Add some frozen fruit—strawberries, peaches, cherries, pineapple, mangos, apricots, blueberries, etc. You can also "start where you are at" by simply using what you have on hand in your refrigerator, freezer, and fruit bowl.

Your green smoothie is the ideal delivery system for additives like spirulina, flaxseed, hemp seed, pumpkin and sunflower seeds, wheat grass, etc. this can be accomplished by adding one or two teaspoons to your smoothie. Or by making milk from hemp, pumpkin, sunflower, sesame, or flax seeds, and using that as a base for your green smoothie.

Experiment and find what works for you. But don't forget to check with your health-care professional before making major changes in your diet.

CHAPTER 23
CHILDREN AND GREEN SMOOTHIES

Green smoothies are an excellent way to get your children to eat fresh fruit and vegetables…and not complain about it.

You can integrate green smoothies into your child's diet as snacks or as lunch. You can serve them as dessert, making them a little heavier on the fruit side for palatability. By rotating your smoothies between breakfast, lunch, dinner, snacks, and dessert, you run interference on your child's singing the boredom blues: "I hate that stuff!"

Getting your children to participate in the process can sometimes go a long way to encouraging them to drink their smoothies. Let them pick a vegetable or fruit that is going to be used. Spell it, let them handle it, let them put it into the blender and talk about how the fruit or veggie grows. And tell them what benefits they'll receive by eating/drinking it.

Whatever you do, don't take forever to create the smoothie. If you take too long between preparation time and drinking time, you'll lose them. The longer you can keep them focused, the better your chances are. Ask their opinion on taste. Is it sweet enough? Does it need more fruit or some honey?

In short, get them involved. Incorporating green smoothies into your child's diet is a creative process. It is a process that you are in control of. Do you want to attach the drinking of green smoothies to nap time, story time, Mummy and me moments, after playtime, as a dessert or a snack? My question to you is, "What does it look like for you to incorporate green smoothies into your child's diet?"

A balanced green smoothie that adheres to the Dietary Principle can be used to supplement and support your child's vitamin intake. As I said earlier, a child's smoothie can be made with a little more fruit than you would normally use. The mantra here is the same: *Start where you are at!*

Another point to remember is that you are in control of what your child does and does not eat. Do not allow your children to dictate what you feed them. If their food of choice is chocolate cake washed down with soda pop, I know you will not be serving this to them for every meal. Why? Because you are making the choice as to what and when they eat.

Here is something that may be helpful for you in the preparation of your child's green smoothies. They are timesaving, cost-effective Little Green Pouches (reusable) or Infantino Squeeze Pouches (disposable). These are empty pouches like the ones that contain pureed fruits and vegetables that kids seem to love; only you fill them yourself. Both are readily available at Amazon.com. They are easy to use. Simply make your green smoothie, fill the pouches, place them in the refrigerator, and whip them out when your child needs a snack, lunch, dinner, and/or dessert. What this also means is that you can ensure that your children are eating what you want them to eat, whether they are at the nursery or on a play date.

If you are wanting your child to have a healthier diet and not use supplements like PediaSure, then you, as the parent, make the choice to change. It's important that you have a plan, and that you are resolute in your intention. Having a plan provides you with clarity that will lend itself to giving you the steps needed to integrate green smoothies into your child's diet. It also provides your child with a safe place and boundaries within which to explore their culinary world.

Garbage in is garbage out. What you are feeding your child today is the foundation of what they will build their health upon for life.

If you are unsure about adding green smoothies to your child's diet, **talk with your pediatrician**.

Q: Can my baby drink green smoothies?

A: If your child is eating solid food, then yes. If your child is drinking milk only, then NO. Be guided by your health-care professional.

Q: Can I use yoghurt in my child's smoothies?

A: Yes, although my suggestion would be to try making them with nut milks.

Q: Will my child get enough vitamin C and protein?

A: Yes. Fruits, vegetables and green leafy vegetables and nuts are packed with protein and vitamins including C.

Q: Can I put my child on a green smoothie fast?

A: No. Not without checking with your child's pediatrician or a health care professional.

Q: Can I use green smoothies to replace a meal?

A: Yes. You can use green smoothies to replace, breakfast, lunch, or dinner.

Q: How do I incorporate green smoothies into my child's dietary lifestyle?

A: You can use green smoothies as a snack or as dessert, or when getting ready for story- or naptime. You can even use your green smoothie as treat of the day. Be creative about how you choose to include them into your child's dietary lifestyle.

CHAPTER 24
WHAT TO DO WHEN IT TASTES WRONG

Occasionally you might create a smoothie that tastes—not so good. It's not horrid enough to be tossed down the garbage disposal, but it's something that you know you'll never make again, even by accident.

I have been asked, "Is there anything that can be done?" I know from experience what it's like. During my 35-day green smoothie fast, I made two green smoothies that were not so good. One was semi-okay after I added agave and organic vanilla extract, and the other was...well, the more I added stuff to make it right the worse it became.

So what can you do when it goes wrong? There are two things that go a long way to making a wrong-tasting smoothie palatable: natural sweeteners and vanilla.

Add a natural sweetener of your choice and a teaspoon of vanilla or half a vanilla bean into the blend will make most "wrong" smoothies taste nearly right. Occasionally, a dash of salt or even a splash of hot sauce or a tiny piece of chili pepper can transform your smoothie.

If nothing you add transforms your smoothie into something that you can get down ...toss it out and start from scratch.

PART THREE

CHAPTER 25
EQUIPMENT

Getting your equipment is really stress-free. You really don't need that much. In fact, to start you only need four things:

1. A blender
2. Something to put your green smoothie in
3. Fruits and vegetables
4. And to, "*Start where you are at!*"

However, to conduct a green smoothie fast and/or include green smoothies into your current dietary practices on a regular basis, the following equipment will be helpful:

Blender (preferably high-powered Vitamix, Blendtec, or Ninja)
4 – 6 Mason jars (32 fl. oz.) with lids
Nut-milk bags (32 fl. oz.) or cheesecloth for straining
Large bowl
A box of straws
Saran Wrap/Cling Film or Press'n Seal
Cutting board
Colander or strainer

Paring knife
Vegetable peeler
Salad spinner
Cooler (traveling)
Ice pack
Vegetable wash
Labels (optional, but useful if making smoothies in advance)

What Do I do With The Press'n Seal/Cling Film/Saran Wrap?

Press'n seal or cling film is used to seal the mouth of your Mason jar or glass. Once the jar has been covered, the cling film is then pierced with a knife, making two small slits. One is for the straw and the other is for airflow to facilitate the drinking of your green smoothie. Covering the mouth of the jar allows you to drink your green smoothie inside or outside without worrying about insects, dust, and pollutants.

Blenders

A blender with a powerful motor is preferable to one with lower horsepower. The more horsepower your blender has, the smoother your green smoothies will be. It is in your best interest to invest in a blender with a powerful motor or greater horsepower for more efficiency when creating your Green Is 4 Life smoothies. It allows the fruits, nuts, and raw vegetables to be blended into a superfine mixture for greater absorption.

However, if your budget doesn't support your purchasing a new or a top-of-the-line blender, simply use what you have or purchase what you can afford. The two adjustments you will have to make are to chop up your fruit and vegetables fairly small and to blend them for much longer. You may have noticed that I included Ninja in the higher horsepower list. This is a good consideration if your budget doesn't support your purchasing a Vitamix or Blendtec. *Start where you are at.*

CHAPTER 26
21 TIPS FOR SUCCESSFULLY ADDING GREEN SMOOTHIES INTO YOUR LIFE

✓ Most green leafy vegetables like spinach, chard, kale, etc. have stems attached, so you don't have to go hunting for stems. (See the Dietary Principle, chapter 7.)

✓ Coconut water when added to your smoothie gives it a turbo boost of vitamins, mineral, trace minerals, electrolytes, etc.

✓ Have what you need on hand.

✓ Plan for the week (or 4/5 days) what green leafy veggies and fruit you want.

✓ Freeze seasonal fruit for later use.

✓ Make your smoothies in advance to support your work schedule.

✓ Green smoothies made in advance will thicken. This is natural. To thin, add water or coconut water and shake well.

✓ Let people know what you are doing, so that when you say, "No, I'm not on the fast food track," they know where you are coming from.

✓ Drink a smoothie while cooking or in a restaurant. (Have Mason jar with green smoothie, will travel.)

✓ Don't fight the craving. If you are craving chocolate, put carob powder or raw chocolate into your smoothie. If you are craving

✓ salt, put a pinch of Celtic salt into your smoothie. If it's sushi, as was my case, add half a sheet of seaweed to your smoothie.

✓ Give into the desire to chew by freezing one of the green smoothie blends you love, or by freezing pureed fruit, or by simply chewing ice. Or make a chunky smoothie.

✓ Come off a green smoothie fast slowly by eating tiny bowls of fruit with a few nuts. Graduate to large bowls and then move to raw vegetables, then steamed, then sautéed, stir-fried, etc.

✓ Purchase a case of 32-ounce Mason jars for adults and 8- or 16-ounce ones for children.

✓ Prewash all vegetable so that they are ready to go when you are. Be sure to dry them well!

✓ Make nut milks in advance. (See recipes in chapter 19.)

✓ Take 32 ounces of water up to bed with you each night. This will bring it to room temperature and it will be the first thing you drink for the day. A twist of lemon or lime is optional.

✓ Get the support you need—reflexology, colonics, massage, coaching, etc.

✓ Know the difference between detoxifying and a medical emergency. If you are unable to tell, seek medical attention.

✓ Purchase fruits and veggies that are within your budget.

✓ Rotate your fruits, nuts, grains, seeds, vegetables, and leafy greens.

✓ First choice is fresh; second choice frozen; third is glass jars.

Start where you are at! The most important consideration is your start point. *Start where you are at.* If you have a blender, fruits, and veggies, and something to drink your smoothie from, you are set.

CHAPTER 27
PANTRY

Here are some ingredients you may want to keep on hand or might like to try.

Green leafy vegetables
Arugula
Beets
Bok choy
Cabbage
Collard greens
Dandelion greens
Kale
Lettuce
Mustard greens
Swiss chard
Spinach
Sorrel
Watercress
Fresh herbs: Basil, dill, mint, rosemary, sage, tarragon, thyme (always use sparingly, one or two leaves)

Vegetables
Asparagus
Avocado

Beets
Broccoli
Brussels sprouts
Carrots
Cauliflower
Celery
Cucumbers
Garlic
Ginger
Green beans
Onions
Parsnips
Peas
Peppers
Radishes
Spring onions
Sprouts
Turnips
Zucchini

Citrus fruits
Grapefruit
Limes
Lemons
Mandarins
Oranges
Sour oranges
Tangelos
Tangerines

Hard-pitted fruits
Cherries
June plums
Mangos

Nectarines
Peaches
Plums

Soursop or Custard apple
Sweetsop or Custard apple

Simple fruits
Apples
Bananas
Berries
Dates
Figs
Grapes
Melons
Pineapples
Tomatoes

Nuts
Almonds
Brazil nuts
Cashews
Coconuts
Hazelnuts
Pecans
Pine nuts
Soybeans
Walnuts

Grains
Barley
Oats
Spelt
Rice

Seeds
Hemp
Pumpkin
Quinoa
Sesame
Sunflower

Liquids
Coconut water—young coconut (not from concentrate or
pasteurized)
Fresh-squeezed juices (not from concentrate or pasteurized)
Kefir water
Spring water

Dairy-plant based
Coconut milk kefir
Coconut yoghurt
Soy yoghurt
Tofu silken

Dairy-milk
Organic yoghurt (low-heat pasteurization)
Organic goats yoghurt
Plain milk kefir

CHAPTER 28
DOS AND DON'TS

Don't have an overly complicated blend, if you use the Dietary Principle, you will not over-create your green smoothie.

Over-creation of your green smoothie is when you have either too much of one thing or too many different things in your blend. It can end up being 'way too earthy, like drinking mud, or too heavy, making you feel bloated. It can even be insipid and totally tasteless. Your Green Is 4 Life Smoothie will, if blended correctly, make your taste buds zing.

Remember, keep it simple: one each of root, stem, leaf, (most leafy vegetables have stems attached) fruit, seeds, and, if desired, herbs. For instance, almond milk (seed), Swiss chard (leaf and stem), parsnips (root), cherries (fruit), plus half a sage leaf. You have the whole plant plus a smattering of an herb. Many of the green leafy vegetables come with lots of stem, but if it's all leaf and hardly any stem, you can always add celery.

Don't drink your green smoothie straight from the refrigerator, allow it to sit at room temperature for about 15 minutes.

Be creative. Think outside your comfort zone. Use avocado in place of banana to achieve that smooth creamy texture. Or try papaya or butternut squash. Use sweet parsnips instead of carrots; try fruits and vegetables that you've never had before. Think outside the jar!

Do take the opportunity to freeze luscious ripe seasonal fruit when available.

Fresh nut, seed and grain milks to be used in your smoothies can be made in advance. (See chapter 19 for nut milk recipes.)

Do make your green smoothies in advance. It is natural for them to thicken. To thin, add water or coconut water and shake well.

Boost your smoothies with coconut water, either from the fresh young coconut or coconut water in the carton, but not from concentrate. (See chapter 8.)

CHAPTER 29
RECIPES

With the variety of fruits, nuts, seeds, vegetables, green leafy vegetables, grains, and nuts available, your choices for making your Green Is 4 Life Smoothies are limitless. All recipes listed make approximately 1 quart, 2 pints or 1 liter.

Honey Do
2 cups coconut water
½ Jazz apple
1 small clove garlic
½ large ripe avocado
2 packed cups collard greens (or greens of your choice)
¼ honeydew melon seeded peeled and cut
1 cup frozen strawberries
Pinch salt (optional)

Blend the first 3 ingredients until the combination looks slushy. Add the other ingredients to blender in order listed and blend until smooth and creamy. *Bon appétit!* You can thin your smoothie out with water or coconut water if it's too thick. If it's too thin, add more fruit, greens, or avocado.

Sunflowers & Peaches
1½ cups coconut water or water
½ Golden Delicious apple

1 small carrot
1 stick celery
¼ lime
1 tbsp. hulled sunflower seeds
1 banana
2 packed cups kale
½ cup strawberries
¼ cup peaches

Blend the first 6 ingredients until they look slushy. Add the other ingredients to blender in order listed and blend until smooth and creamy. *Bon appétit!* You can thin your smoothie out with water or coconut water if it's too thick. If it's too thin, add more fruit, greens, or avocado.

Orange, Papaya, & Mint
1½ cups coconut water or water
1 small carrot
1 Pink Lady apple
¼ peeled cucumber
¼ - ½ papaya
3 cups spinach
2-4 large mint leaves
2 peeled frozen oranges
½ cup frozen peaches

Blend the first 4 ingredients until they look slushy. Add the other ingredients to blender in order listed and blend until smooth and creamy. *Bon appétit.* You can thin your smoothie out with water or coconut water if it's too thick. If it's too thin, add more fruit, greens, tofu or avocado.

Cherry Kale Chocolate
11/2 cups hazelnut milk (See nut milk recipes.)
¼ peeled cucumber
1 banana
3 cups kale
1-cup cherries

Blend all ingredients until smooth and creamy. This taste like chocolate! You can thin your smoothie out with water or coconut water if it's too thick. If it's too thin, add more fruit, greens, or avocado.

Almond Basil Surprise
1½ cups almond milk
1 small carrot
1 green apple
1 banana
¼ cantaloupe, peeled and seeded
1 bunch Swiss chard
½ cup strawberries
½ cup peaches

Blend the first 3 ingredients until slushy. Add the other ingredients to blender in order listed and blend until smooth and creamy. *Bon appétit.* You can thin your smoothie out with water or coconut water if it's too thick. If it's too thin, add more fruit, greens, or avocado.

Brazilian Mango
11/2 cups Brazil nut milk sweetened with Medjool dates or sweetener of choice
½ peeled zucchini (courgette)
1 slice sweet potato (yam) or ½ red or golden beet
1 large ripe mango, peeled, with stone removed
2 cups greens
1 handful dandelion greens
½ cup frozen peaches

Blend the first 3 ingredients until slushy. Add the other ingredients to blender in order listed and blend until smooth and creamy. *Bon appétit.* You can thin your smoothie out with water or coconut water if it's too thick. If it's too thin, add more fruit, greens, or avocado.

Coconut Lime
2 cups coconut water or coconut milk

½ cup white grapes
1 stick celery
¼ organic lime with peel
1 banana
1/8 honeydew
2 cups bok choy
¾ cup frozen strawberries

Blend the first 4 ingredients until slushy. Add the other ingredients to blender in order listed and blend until smooth and creamy. *Bon appétit.*

You can thin your smoothie out with water or coconut water if it's too thick. If it's too thin, add more fruit, greens, or avocado.

Apricot Delight
2 cups cashew nut milk
1 carrot
½ peeled cucumber
1 pear
1 banana
½ cup ripe apricots
3 cups spinach or sorrel
6 green beans
¾ cups strawberries

Blend the first 4 ingredients until slushy. Add the other ingredients to blender in order listed and blend until smooth and creamy. *Bon appétit.*

You can thin your smoothie out with water or coconut water if it's too thick. If it's too thin, add more fruit, greens, or avocado.

Parsnip Delight
2 cups cashew nut milk, sweetened with Medjool dates (See nut milk recipes.)
1 small parsnip, peeled and cut into chunks
1 banana
1 bunch Swiss chard
1 cup strawberries

Blend the first 2 ingredients until fairly smooth. Add the other ingredients to blender in order listed and blend until smooth and creamy. *Bon appétit.*

You can thin your smoothie out with water or coconut water if it's too thick. If it's too thin, add more fruit, greens, or avocado.

Fruit Explosion
1½ cup coconut water
1 apple or pear
1¼- inch slice celery root
1 teaspoon golden flax seed
1 banana or silken tofu
3 cups mixed greens—baby Swiss chard (green and red) and baby spinach
¼ cup blueberries
¼ cup cherries
½ cup peaches

Blend the first 4 ingredients until slushy. Add the other ingredients to blender in order listed and blend until smooth and creamy. *Bon appétit.* You can thin your smoothie out with water or coconut water if it's too thick. If it's too thin, add more fruit, greens, or avocado.

Chocoholic
2 cups coconut milk
2 tbsp. carob powder or raw chocolate powder
½ vanilla pod or ½ tsp. vanilla extract
1 Asian pear
½ icicle radish or 1 red radish
½ avocado or banana
2 cups sorrel or spinach
½ cup black cherries

Blend the first 5 ingredients until slushy. Add the other ingredients to blender in order listed and blend until smooth and creamy. *Bon appétit.*

You can thin your smoothie out with water or coconut water if it's too thick. If it's too thin, add more fruit, greens, or avocado.

Pineapple Treat
2 cups coconut water
1 cup pineapple, fresh or frozen
½ cucumber
½ parsnip
1 banana
3 cups yellow Swiss chard or green Swiss chard
½ cup peaches

Blend the first 4 ingredients until slushy. Add the other ingredients to blender in order listed and blend until smooth and creamy. *Bon appétit.*

You can thin your smoothie out with water or coconut water if it's too thick. If it's too thin, add more fruit, greens, or avocado.

Romaine Strawberry Salad
2 cups water or coconut water
¼ lime
1 apple
1 asparagus spear
¼ zucchini
1 carrot
1 banana or ½ avocado
6 large romaine lettuce leaves
1 cup dandelion leaves
2 basil leaves
¾ cup strawberries

Blend the first 6 ingredients until slushy. Add the other ingredients to blender in order listed and blend until smooth and creamy. *Bon appétit.*

You can thin your smoothie out with water or coconut water if it's too thick. If it's too thin, add more fruit, greens, or avocado.

Spicy Veggie Roll Smoothie
2 - 4 cups water or coconut water

1 carrot
1 apple
1/8 lime
¼ red bell pepper
¼ cucumber
1 sliver serrano pepper
½ - 1 large, ripe avocado
1 peeled ripe kiwi
2 bok choy leaves
1 cup spinach
1 basil leaf
1 mint leaf
1 cup frozen grapes or peaches
Pinch Celtic salt (optional)

Blend the first 7 ingredients until slushy. Add the other ingredients to blender in order listed and blend until smooth and creamy. *Bon appétit.*

You can thin your smoothie out with water or coconut water if it's too thick. If it's too thin, add more fruit, greens, or avocado.

Sun Showers
2 cups sunflower seed milk sweetened with dates or sweetener of your choice
½ small parsnip
1 Jazz or Pink Lady apple
½ stick celery
¼ vanilla bean
1 banana
2 cups spinach
1 cup dandelion greens
5 mint leaves
1 cup frozen strawberries

Blend the first 5 ingredients until slushy. Add the other ingredients to blender in order listed and blend until smooth and creamy. *Bon appétit.*

You can thin your smoothie out with water or coconut water if it's too thick. If it's too thin, add more fruit or greens.

Baby Steps
2 cups water or coconut water
6 green beans or 3 pieces green vegetable of your choice
1 mango
½ cup pineapple
1 banana

Blend the first 2 ingredients until slushy. Add the other ingredients to blender in order listed and blend until smooth and creamy. *Bon appétit.*

You can thin your smoothie out with water or coconut water if it's too thick. If it's too thin, add more fruit, greens, or avocado.

Also, silken Tofu, an excellent source of plant protein can be used as a substitute for banana or avocado to thicken your green smoothie. Remember tofu has no flavor and takes on the flavor of what it's paired with.

Be creative with your green smoothie blends. It's your life; it's your choice. *Bon appétit.*

CHAPTER 30
CONCLUSION

Your life is built upon the choices you make. Each choice represents the life that you have built and the life that you are currently building. Part of that building process surrounds what you eat. In fact, food is central to many cultures and is an integral part of our socialization and expression. You are what you eat. This axiom is fact and not merely an old adage.

Green smoothies are a perfect fit. No matter where you are in the world, if there is plant life and water you can create a smoothie. You don't even need a blender. A large mortar and pestle, with a little muscle power, will do just as well.

Green smoothies are not a panacea. However, they are nature's medicine in the form of food. And a green smoothie created with fresh green leafy vegetables, other vegetables, sun-ripened fruits, nuts, seeds, and grains is an ideal delivery system for essential nutrients that the body requires to maintain and sustain optimal health.

The nutrients found in green leafy vegetables, other vegetables, ripe fruits, nuts, seeds, and grains include proteins, minerals, trace minerals, vitamins, fiber, and water. They also carry the vital life force that is in every living thing. These elements are essential for triggering our innate healing response for healthy cell renewal.

Green smoothies also offer a sustainable and renewable source of food that is eco-friendly or "green." Nature has provided us with a wide variety of vegetation, which allows each individual, I believe, the right, to choose what is best for "self."

Green smoothies by design are all about the inclusion of raw life-giving vegetables and fruits. Adding green smoothies into your life is not about the exclusion of the things that you love to eat. You have the power to change your life by choosing to include this delicious and nutritious drink into your life. You will be amazed by the results. It's not just your health that will be positively impacted, but your wealth, your relationships and your self-expression.

Food really is nature's finest medicine and is worthy of your serious consideration and exploration. Green smoothies are the vital life force of plants, captured in a jar, blended in an efficient way that makes this energetic healing force easy to consume for optimum absorption.

If we are what we eat, then the question that begs to be asked is "What are you eating?"

CHAPTER 31
RESOURCES

There are several resources that were influential in helping me to make my decision to conduct a 35-day green smoothie fast, a choice that has irrevocably changed my life. Below is a list of some resources you may want to explore.

Movies/Documentaries
Fat, Sick & Nearly Dead
Directed by Joe Cross, Kurt Engfehr. Us & Us Media, 2010, Warner Bros., 2011

Hungry for Change
Directed by James Colquhoun, Laurentine Ten Bosch. Permacology Productions, 2012

Food, Inc. Directed by Robert Kenner. Magnolia Home Entertainment, 2009

Farmageddon
Directed by Kristen Canty. Gravitas Ventures LLC, 2011

The Gerson Miracle
Directed by Steve Kroschel. Cinema Libre, 2009

Books
Blythman, Joanna
What to Eat: Food That's Good for Your Health, Pocket and Plate
London, Fourth Estate, 2012

Cabot, Sandra M.D. *The Juice Fasting Bible*
Berkeley CA, Ulysses Press, 2007

Dale, Cindi
New Chakra Healing
St Paul, MN, Llewellyn Publications, 1996

Kloss, Jethro
Back To Eden
Twin Lakes, WI, Lotus Press, 1939-2002

Miles, Kristine
The Green Smoothie Bible
Berkeley CA, Ulysses Press, 2012

Pollan, Michael
Food Rules: An Eater's Manual
New York, NY, Penguin Books, 2009

Reid, Lori
Color Book
London, Connections Book Publishing, 2000

Websites
All About Fasting
Egyptian and Fasting Quotes
http://www.allaboutfasting.com/fasting-quotes.html

British Red
The Science of Fire, 2.1 Understanding Fuel
http://www.orionn49.com

The Science of how stuff works
Why Does Smoke Come From Fire?
http://science.howstuffworks.com/environmental/energy/question43.htm

Questions, Suggestions & Recipes

For questions concerning you and your green smoothie experience, please contact me via email
drwendy@itsmylifemychoice.com

To share recipes and tips please go to the forum
http://www.itsmylifemychoice.com/green-is-4-life-smoothies

About The Author

Dr. Wendy Dearborne is the founder of, "It's My Life My Choice." She is an author, lecturer, choice expert and holistic health practitioner. Through the power of personal *conscious choice* she supports people who are seeking permanent healthy lifestyle changes, by giving tools that are simple and easily integrated into any lifestyle.

A life changing personal experience, altered the trajectory of her life and catapulted her on a spiritual journey that lead to the discovery that, "our lives are created one choice at a time." Her passion is to use her personal and professional expertise to deliver this message to all who will embrace it.

Dr. Wendy has a weekly internet radio talk show called "My Life My Choice, which is focused on providing her listening audience choice making tools. She was born and raised in Tottenham, North London and now makes her home, with her husband Dee, in Las Vegas, Nevada.

Email:	Drwendy@itsmylifemychoice.com
Websites:	http://www.itsmylifemychoice.com
	http://www.drwendydearborne.com

My Life My Choice
Dr. Wendy's weekly internet radio show. Live Wednesday's at 1.00pm. Archived episodes available. Podcasts available from iTunes.
http://www.blogtalkradio.com/mylifemychoice